Firm Loose Skin
A Guide to Natural and Effective Non-Surgical Skin Tightening Methods

Firm Loose Skin
A Guide to Natural and Effective Non-Surgical Skin Tightening Methods

Melynda Majors

All rights reserved.

No part of this book may be reproduced in any form or by any means, including scanning, photocopying or otherwise, without prior written permission of the copyright holder except where otherwise noted within the book. Brief passages may be excerpted for review.

Copyright © 2012 by Melynda Majors
Printed in the United States of America
First Edition

ISBN 14-8005-729-0
ISBN-13 978-1-48-005729-6

Special thanks to Basil Tilmon.

Disclaimer and Terms of Use

The Author and Publisher have attempted to be as accurate and complete as possible in the writing and publishing of this book. The content of this book is not and cannot be warranted. While all possible attempts have been made to verify information provided in this book, the Author and Publisher assume no responsibility for errors, omissions or contrary interpretation of the subject matter within.

This book contains general information about medical conditions and treatments. The information presented in this book is provided for educational and informational purposes only, is not intended as medical advice, and should not be treated as such. The Author is not a medical doctor, registered dietician, or clinical nutritionist. No health claims are made by this book. The information contained in this book is not to be used to diagnose or treat or cure any illness, disorder, disease, medical condition, health problem or any other issue. Readers are urged to seek the advice of trained medical personnel on a regular basis and before implementing any of the suggestions in this book. Always consult your physician or health care provider before beginning any nutrition or exercise program. Use of the programs, advice, and information contained in this book is at the sole choice and risk of the reader. No warranty is given or implied.

The Author and Publisher shall have neither liability nor responsibility to any person or entity with respect to any of the information contained in this book. The reader assumes any and all risk for any injury, loss or damage caused or alleged to be caused, directly or indirectly by accessing and/or using any information described in this book. The Author and Publisher make no representations or warranties in relation to the information in this book, express or implied.

The Author and Publisher do not warrant that the information contained in this book is complete, true, accurate, up-to-date, or non-misleading. Do not rely on the information in this book or indeed in any book as an alternative to medical advice from your doctor or other professional health care provider. If you have any specific questions about any medical matter or health concern you should consult your doctor or other health care professional. If you think you may be suffering from any medical condition you should seek immediate medical attention. You should never delay seeking medical advice, disregard medical advice, or discontinue medical treatment because of information in this book. Nothing in this medical disclaimer will limit any of our liabilities in any way that is not permitted under applicable law, or exclude any of our liabilities that may not be excluded under applicable law. Any perceived slights of specific persons, products or organizations are unintentional.

All the beauty of the world, 'tis but skin deep.
                                        -Ralph Venning, 1650

For Amanda, Daulton, David, Herman,
John, Leon, Linda and Shannon,
          with love.

Contents

Foreword		xiii
Introduction		xvi
1	What Is Skin and Why Does It Sag?	1
2	Loose Skin or Loose Fat?	6
3	Tighten Skin From the Inside Out and From the Outside In: Superfoods, Supplements and External Treatments	11
	Skin-Tightening Substances, Vitamin A to Zinc	17
	Treatments by Target	46
	Recommended Daily Allowances	48
	Skin-Tightening Internal Supplements	53
	Skin-Tightening Cremes, Lotions, Oils and External Treatments Ingredients	54
	Skin-Tightening Superfoods	55
4	Skin-Tightening Exercises	61
	Build a Firm Foundation With Heavy Lifting	62
	Rebounding	65
	Foam Roller Exercises	68
	Working Out From the Neck Up	68
5	Other Non-Surgical Treatments	72
	Dry-Skin Brushing	73
	Non-Surgical Cosmetic Procedures	74
	Detoxification	75
	Compression Garments	78
6	Real-Life Skin-Tightening Stories	80
7	Summary: *What Now?*	86

Afterword: Looking Like a Basset Hound,
    Good or Bad?   89

References and Resources for Further
    Reading   91

About the Author   140

Final Thoughts   141

Foreword

I have struggled with my weight my entire life. When I was a baby, so my mother tells me, I would squall at the end of my first bottle if I wasn't immediately given a second.

My first clear memory of being ashamed of my weight was when I was eight years old. My mother took me to the local hospital for a fasting blood sugar test to check for diabetes. At the time, I already weighed over 100 pounds and was significantly larger than my classmates. I wasn't yet obese, but I was definitely overweight.

My weight increased each year and I weighed well over 250 pounds by eleventh grade. As I entered my senior year in high school, I decided to take matters into my own hands and I began taking an over-the-counter appetite suppressant—I think it was Dexatrim—while basically starving myself. I remember one week I ate three pieces of fried chicken—that was my entire food intake for the week.

This regimen was stupid and dangerous, but it worked. By the time I graduated from high school I had dropped to around 175 pounds—certainly not small for my height of 5'8, but on the high end of normal.

I maintained that weight for two years by starving and taking aerobics classes in college. By my junior year of college I had moved away from home to my first apartment and my eating immediately got out of control. I gained and gained and gained. I went from a size 16 to an 18 to a 20, where I stayed for a year or two. Then, a couple of years out of college, I began gaining again and ultimately, by the time I was 30 years old, I wore a size 28 at over 300 pounds.

In 1999 I discovered dieting through carbohydrate restriction (the Atkins Diet) and I quickly dropped 100 pounds, going from a size 28 to a size 16. I looked and felt great.

But life intervened, I slacked off from dieting, and all those hard-lost pounds returned—with friends. By 2004, I weighed more than ever and I looked and felt terrible—fat, old, depressed, miserable and in pain. Going up and down stairs was pure torture on my feet, legs and knees.

In 2008 I rediscovered low-carb and, from a starting weight of 370, lost all the weight again. I have maintained my new smaller size for nearly five years and I continue to lose slowly but steadily. I've been through stalls and setbacks but I haven't regained. I look and feel much, much better—younger, healthier, more energetic. It's wonderful.

But gaining and losing and gaining and losing weight multiple times has not been kind to my skin. When I re-dedicated myself to losing weight in 2008, I was very concerned about the possibility of getting to a normal weight but being burdened with saggy, excess skin. Part of me thought, what was the point of going to the trouble to lose all this weight if I'm going to look like a saggy, droopy basset hound?

I was determined to lose weight anyway and to worry about possible loose skin later. Well, "later" has arrived—and with it, loose skin. Lots of it. The search for a solution to my own problem with loose skin led me to research the heck out of the topic and ultimately to write this book.

I have spent the last few years compiling, analyzing and testing (to the extent possible for a non-scientist) natural remedies for sagging skin. I have not written this book as a scientific researcher or a medical doctor. I am neither. I have written it as a fellow sufferer who happens to be a strong researcher, as someone who understands first-hand the issue of loose skin, and as someone who has spent many hours trying to piece together the most likely natural, non-surgical remedies. If you're going through what I'm going through with my loose skin, I hope my research, which led to this book, can help both of us tighten our skin without resorting to surgical intervention.

Read this book using your own common sense. If a proposed solution sounds practical and doable to you and your doctor, try it. Nothing in this book should harm you if you are otherwise healthy, not pregnant or nursing, and not on any prescription or other medications. But *please* get your doctor's OK before making any changes to your personal health care regimen, including implementing any suggestions proposed in this book.

Plastic surgery is an option for many people with loose skin, but for others, it's not. You may be concerned about the dangers of surgery, the pain and the difficulty of post-surgical recovery. Your health insurance may not pay for plastic surgery and you may not be able to afford it on your own. That doesn't mean your loose skin situation is hopeless.

Read this book. Implement any suggestions you feel drawn to. And keep a positive attitude!

Many people who have lost significant amounts of weight or who have given birth to very large babies that have stretched out their skin report that skin does firm naturally over time, all by itself.

The suggestions in this book are meant to help this process along, to speed it up as much as possible, to give us hope, and, ultimately, to reduce or even eliminate the need for surgical intervention altogether, if possible.

Let's take this journey together!

Introduction

When I recommitted to a low-carb lifestyle in 2008 I joined a number of diet-related Internet discussion forums and web boards. And from that day to this, one of the hottest topics on every forum I belong to is the fear of loose, saggy skin after weight loss. "Newbies," people new to the board or new to dieting, frequently post questions regarding the possibility of loose skin after losing weight. Basically, they seek the community's assurance that their skin will remain taught, or tighten up quickly and naturally, during and after weight loss.

The most common response seems to be—no one knows. Post-weight loss skin firmness seems to hinge on a number of factors, including age, highest weight, length of time spent at highest weight, genetic factors and, some say, speed of weight loss. Personally, I don't believe speed of weight loss affects skin taughtness to a great extent. I believe that, if a person needs to lose weight, their health is best served by losing it as quickly as their doctor advises. Put your overall health first and other considerations, such as loose skin, second.

But, if someone develops loose skin during or after weight loss, as an aftermath of pregnancy, years of tanning or due to simple aging, is plastic surgery the only solution? Or is natural skin tightening possible? The answer varies from person to person but this book compiles the best and most effective methods I've been able to find, as well as other proposed solutions, to loose skin.

If you're looking for the "magic answer," or an instant solution, then that's probably going to be plastic surgery. But if you're not yet ready for plastic surgery, if you're worried about the potential side effects, the potential pain, the danger inherent in any surgical procedure or the expense—or if you simply prefer to try a natural solution first—keep reading. There is hope.

Chances are, many of the items recommended in this book already are in your refrigerator or medicine cabinet. Maybe your're like me, you've spent time in the beauty aisle trying to figure out which lotions to try to firm up your skin, and you've walked away more confused and frustrated than before you started. Maybe friends have recommended weird exercises, or jogging, or toning with light weights, and you're frustrated because nothing you've tried so far has worked. And, if you're too impatient to read the entire book I have summarized all the key findings in the Summary. It's OK to skip ahead.

I'm glad you're reading this book, and I invite you to join me on this journey to firmer, tighter skin.

Finally, I encourage you to send me your own skin-tightening story through this book's website, at www.firmlooseskin.com. Has one of the methods in this book worked or failed for you? Please share your story so we can all benefit. You can contact me through the website and I would love to hear your story of what works and what doesn't work, for you.

1

What Is Skin and Why Does it Sag?

Skin is the largest organ of the human body and it is the key component of the integumentary system, which also includes hair and nails. Its job is to protect the human body, to accept sensations from external stimuli giving us our sense of touch, to excrete waste through oil and perspiration, and to regulate temperature, among other things.

Skin has layers. The outer layer is the epidermis; below that is the dermis. The dermis consists of dense irregular connective tissue, hair follicles, sweat glands, blood vessels, lymph vessels and other things. The dermis layer gives skin its elasticity and it is the key player in the fight against wrinkling and sagging; two of its key components are collagen and elastin. Collagen makes connective tissue strong; elastin, as the name implies, makes it elastic.

Connective tissue is made up of cells in an extracellular matrix which consists of fibers and ground substance. The cells making up connective tissue include adipocytes, fibroblasts, lymphocytes, macrophages, mast cells and other cells. The fibers helping to hold this all together include collagen fibers, elastic fibers and reticular fibers. Adipocytes store fat. Fibroblasts secrete the fibers and ground substance of the extracellular matrix. Lymphocytes, circulating via the lymph system, are involved in immune defense and inflammation. Macrophages remove damaged cells and other foreign materials. Mast cells also trigger inflammation.

Fibroblasts are the most common of these cells found in connective tissue. They secrete collagen and they are essential for normal connective tissue development and repair. They heal wounds to the skin and they are what form scars during tissue repair. Scars are comprised of collagen deposited by fibroblasts when repairing tissue damage. Microphages digest the excretions of other cells. They are mobile over short distances within localized areas of connective tissue. Mast cells are triggered to release chemicals creating inflammation when needed–for example, as a response to disease or injury.

Below the dermis lies the hypodermis, which attaches the skin to muscle and bone through loose connective tissue and elastin, and which houses adipose–body fat.

Adipose tissue, or subcutaneous fat, is made up of adipocytes–fat cells. It acts as our body's fuel depot by reserving fat as potential energy for later use and as insulation to keep us warm. Adipocytes store lipid (fat) as reserve energy for our bodies. Each cell contains a single fat droplet surrounded by a thin layer of cell cytoplasm.

Cellulite is a condition whereby excess adipose tissue, typically distributed around the abdomen, buttocks, thighs and legs, takes on a lumpy, orange peel- or cottage cheese-type appearance. Cellulite can have many causes, including gender (primarily female), age, genetic predisposition, and circulatory or lymphatic insufficiency.

The lymph system, which circulates lymphocytes, is one of the most important, and in some ways least known, systems of the human body. In it, lymph vessels carry lymph fluid towards the heart. Lymph can transport bacteria to the lymph nodes, where they may be destroyed, and transports fats from the digestive system. The lymph system also includes the spleen, thymus, lymph nodes and tonsils. The condition of the lymph system is a key diagnostic aid in many conditions, and a well-functioning lymph system is critical to good health.

The heart pumps blood through your cardiovascular system but gravity and daily movement, including exercise, normally pumps lymph fluid through your lymph system. And it's easy for your lymph system to drain sluggishly.

Some people experience unusual problems with their lymph systems. For example, if you experience repeated, sustained swelling in your legs and ankles, this could be a condition called lymphedema. It often is experienced by overweight people and it can be passed down from generation to generation. I inherited this from my mother, she from her mother, and my ankles, feet and legs have swelled off and on since I was in college. For others, it can be a side effect following cancer treatment.

Left untreated, serious cases of lymphedema can result in permanent swelling or worse–like cellulitis, an ulcerated bacterial skin infection which is painful, unsightly and can become permanent. Of course, if you have any of these symptoms or conditions, you should consult your physician because treatment is available. And if you don't, great! I'm not including this to frighten you, but to stress the point that the condition of your lymph system is a very important part of your overall health.

A healthy lymph system is critical to healthy skin and we want to ensure that our skin is as healthy as possible to support it in firming up. One method to improve skin health through lymph system health is dry skin brushing, which many claim not only stimulates the lymph system but also reduces cellulite–it's a great activity to engage in whether you're at goal weight, just beginning a weight loss journey, or anywhere in between. See section five for an introduction to dry skin brushing.

Strengthening and, if needed, healing our lymph system can improve our skin which can help in visibly reducing cellulite. A healthy, well-functioning lymph system is critical to healthy skin and a badly functioning lymph system directly contributes to a host of conditions including, among other things, skin problems.

Many factors can cause your skin to lose its natural elasticity and sag a little, or a lot. Sun tanning can contribute to sagging skin, as can smoking, dehydration, pregnancy and weight loss. Skin also loses natural firmness as it ages.

When you don't protect your skin from excessive sun exposure, or if you overdo it at the tanning bed, your skin can suffer. Photoaging, as it's called by dermatologists, may cause many unwanted changes to the skin including freckles, wrinkles and dryness. Skin cancer also is a serious concern. Years of excessive sun tanning may cause skin to become leathery and loose. If your skin is in this condition from tanning, please consult a dermatologist for a specialized treatment plan.

Smoking has many negative side effects and it is detrimental to your health. It also can have a very negative impact on your skin's elasticity. Lack of adequate hydration, particularly over time, can negatively affect your skin. Further, when a woman's abdomen stretches to accommodate new life, her skin may not snap back to its original firmness after the baby's birth. Losing weight, losing large amounts of weight you've carried for a long time, and/or yo-yoing from high weight to low and back again multiple times can wreak havoc on your skin. It certainly hasn't helped mine at all.

Aging or damaged skin loses collagen and elastin. Collagen, introduced above, is a protein produced by fibroblasts, is the primary component of connective tissue and it is the most common protein in the human body. It is an essential structural element of connective tissues' extracellular matrices and it provides structure, toughness and tensile strength. Scars are made up of collagen. Elastin, also a protein, helps skin retain its shape and regain its shape after distortion. It is a component of the elastic fibers that also help make up connective tissue.

Another enemy to firm skin we should know about are free radicals. Free radicals are highly charged oxygen molecules that are missing an electron. Free radicals in your body steal an electron from other molecules in your body, potentially damaging an otherwise healthy molecule. They are harmful to the skin as well as to the entire human body. They can be brought about by tanning, smoking, chemical exposure, excess body weight and other factors. They damage the skin through causing wrinkling and sagging.

With these skin enemies (let's call them skinemies) coming at us from all sides, it's really no wonder that, as we age, skin that is naturally firm and taught will sag simply due to the ravages of time, not to mention all the other problems we throw at it.

The recommendations in this book are suitable for anyone with sagging skin, regardless of the initial cause. However, you will notice as your read that I'm primarily going to focus on people whose skin sags due to weight loss because this is the background I come to the topic from.

It doesn't matter if your skin is sagging due to having kids, tanning, smoking, poor nutrition, aging or any other reason. The suggestions in this book apply equally whether you're young or old, thin or fat, smooth or wrinkly, pale or leathery. It's never too late to start taking the best care of your skin you can–your skin will thank you, and you and your skin will start to look younger, smoother and firmer before you know it.

This book's premise, and its approach to tightening loose skin by treating plastic surgery as a last resort, not a first resort, lies in:

- helping our bodies build the collagen and elastin they need to strengthen our connective tissue, which is the substance our bodies use to connect skin to muscle;
- improving the lymph system which, when it functions properly, supports healthy skin;
- melting any remaining fat and cellulite that's keeping our skin loose and saggy;
- building the strong muscle foundation our skin needs to adhere to; and,
- improving the external appearance of the skin itself.

We will examine the best science in these areas and come up with a plan of attack to melt any remaining fat and cellulite and to give our skin, our muscles, our connective tissue and our lymph systems every means of support they need to do the job they were designed to do–reconnect our loose skin to our underlying muscle.

2

Loose Skin or Loose Fat?

I'm going to go out on a limb and say, if you're reading this book, chances are you have loose skin—or do you? How can you tell the difference between loose skin and loose fat?

The average thickness of human skin is about 1/10th of an inch. That's it. If you have looseness on your body and it's significantly thicker than 2/10ths of an inch—it's probably loose skin *and* loose fat.

A panniculus is the medical term for a hanging lower belly—essentially, an apron of skin. Plastic surgery typically can remove a panniculus, liposuction out remaining fat and stitch abdominal muscles back together. Some call this a tummy tuck or a "mommy makeover." A brachioplasty, or arm lift, can repair hanging skin on the upper arms and a thighplasty can do the same for thighs and buttocks. The goal of this book is to help us incorporate natural methods to greatly reduce, or, for some, to eliminate the need for these surgical procedures or any other skin-tightening surgeries.

Obviously, our skin stretches as we grow. The volume of skin on an infant is far less than that of an adult. Skin grows, and it also can shrink. We've all seen heartbreaking photos of starving people, and on many you can easily see the outline of their bones through their skin as it shrinks. Skin is amazingly resilient. Again, we've all experienced cuts and scrapes, minor and major. Your skin has the ability to self repair. It's a living organ and it can adapt.

Our first responsibility when beginning a skin-tightening regimen while losing weight is to shed as much remaining fat on our bodies as possible. The amounts we need to lose are as individual as we are, but the more we can safely and healthfully lose, the better our end result will be. Our skin wants to shrink up and adhere to muscle tissue, not fat. So the fat needs to get out the way to allow this to happen. We've all heard the (misleading) saying, "muscle weighs more than fat." A more accurate way to say that is, for the same weight, muscle takes up a lot less space than fat.

What we may think of as "hanging skin" on our upper arms, thighs, buttocks, back, abdomen, chin, neck or anywhere else may very well be hanging fat and/or cellulite in cellulite-prone areas. If you pinch the hanging skin and it's more than a few millimeters thick, again, it's probably hanging skin and fat.

Hanging skin will be very, very thin. It probably will be wrinkly in texture. Skin that is lumpy or cottage cheesy in texture is cellulite–adipose tissue, which is fat, not skin. Reducing your body fat percentage or BMI (body mass index, a method of calculating body fat percentage based on height and weight) is necessary because our skin wants to adhere to muscle, not to fat.

A simple, common-sense way to judge whether we have loose skin or loose fat is to see whether it jiggles. Skin doesn't jiggle, just fat. Jump up and down, wiggle around. If it jiggles, it's fat that needs to be dieted off. If it flaps, it's probably loose skin. Is it lumpy, resembling cottage cheese? Cellulite, not loose skin. Losing weight is the number-one way to reduce cellulite, but other treatments exist and they are closely examined later in the book.

Do we need to wait until we reach goal weight and have a low BMI before we begin tightening our skin? Absolutely not! We will see results closer to what we want to see the closer to goal weight we are. But that does *not* mean we have to wait until we reach goal weight before trying the suggestions in this book. What we do *now* to improve our skin firmness should have an ameliorating effect on skin looseness as we continue to diet, and it will make our connective tissue, muscles and lymph system that much readier to work *for* us when we reach goal weight.

What's the best way to shed that excess weight? The best way is whatever way works for you. Every diet isn't right for every person. Whatever diet you choose to follow must, however, be sustainable. Some diets work for many, many diets work for some. In order to lose weight and keep it off, your diet solution needs to be sustainable over the long haul and you need to think of it as a permanent lifestyle change rather than a temporary solution.

When I was younger I always thought that I could diet down to goal weight then go back to "normal" eating and nature would take care of the rest. Well, for that to succeed, there has to be a new definition of "normal," as I learned the hard way after regaining over 100 pounds twice in my life.

Most diets either incorporate some method of counting (calories, carbs, etc.) and/or restriction (reducing fat or carbs, eliminating certain types of foods and beverages, and so on). Many also incorporate exercise with dieting, which is a good idea as long as your doctor approves. To keep off the weight you've lost or are planning to lose, you simply aren't going to be able to go back to the lifestyle that caused you to gain weight and to be overweight in the first place.

I believe the single best diet is whatever diet works best for you. I have many friends who've lost weight by joining a commercial program like Weight Watchers or Jenny Craig, by counting calories, by counting carbs, and through weight loss surgery. Any of these can be an effective tool if followed properly and in partnership with your health care provider.

But, speaking as someone who's lost nearly 200 pounds and who's kept it off for more than four years now, whatever plan you choose has to resonate with you, you have to love it (or at least make your peace with it), and you have to commit to it and adhere to it, or to some form of it, *for life*.

Losing weight is hard and maintenance truly does not take care of itself. It's so easy to gain weight back. And yo-yoing from high weight to low weight back to high weight back to low weight (like I have) is not going to do your skin or more importantly your overall health any favors.

Choose your plan based on your personal preferences, on what you feel is sustainable for life, and with the advice of your doctor, nutritionist or health care provider.

Keep in mind that you can't spot reduce, unfortunately.

If overall you're still overweight and you're pretty happy with how you look except for the one or two areas which you think may have loose skin—I'm sorry, but I can't give you a magic solution to take weight off just in those areas. Or, to be specific, I can't give you a magic *non-surgical* solution. Probably what you're going to want to consider is liposuction and plastic surgery. And if that's the route you want to go, more power to you. Do what's right for you.

If you're looking solely for a non-surgical technique, however, you're going to need to shed the rest of that weight and get down to a healthy BMI in order for that remaining fat and cellulite to get lost. Many, many people have said that the really stubborn areas don't clear up until the last five-to-ten pounds comes off.

I lost weight, kept it off, and I am still losing on a low-carb diet, but I definitely wouldn't advise everyone to go low carb. It's very restrictive and it can be difficult for carb-lovers to maintain over the long haul. Fortunately, I love protein and fat, and although I miss carbs sometimes, I have made my peace with low-carb and the results keep me motivated and happy.

Choose the plan that's right for you, follow it, believe in it, love it (or at least, don't hate it!), and make it a lifestyle change. Lose the weight you need to lose and use this book as a tool along the way to help your skin snap back as much as it can.

And once you get to goal weight, continue to use this book as long as you need to, until your skin has tightened up as much as you want it to, or until you and your doctor decide it's time to consider plastic surgery. But I believe plastic surgery should be your last resort, not your first, and you probably agree, or you wouldn't be reading this book.

The suggestions presented in this book are intended to reduce or eliminate the need for skin surgery but everyone is different and, as with many things, there are no absolutes. If you adhere to the suggestions that resonate most strongly with you, they should at the very least improve the condition of your loose skin. And the more approaches you take, the better your results should be.

But at some point some of us may decide that non-surgical skin tightening is not enough on its own. If that's the case, following the suggestions in this book should get you at least part of the way there, so any surgeries you decide to have may be far less drastic and invasive than they would have been had you not followed any of this book's suggestions.

Try the methods in this book that appeal to you. Keep an open mind, and commit wholeheartedly to any course of action you decide to follow. And, keep in mind, improving our skin and our connective tissue *is* possible. If you're interested in the science, check the references section at the end of this book for a selection of useful scientific articles.

Now, on to the good stuff—practical, natural, inexpensive and effective non-surgical solutions to help us help our skin bounce back. Let's get ready for bikini season!

3

Tighten Skin From the Inside Out and From the Outside In: Superfoods, Supplements and External Treatments

Once thought to be un-repairable, connective tissue is now known to be able to recover and heal from injury. Scientific evidence now supports the idea that nutritional therapy is a key factor in repairing connective tissue. It's important to take in nutrition–either through supplements or as they naturally occur in foods, assuming the foods are permitted on any diet you may happen to be following–that concentrates on supporting and repairing connective tissue, skin, muscles and the lymph system.

The key to firming our skin is to repair our connective tissue, our overall skin health and our lymph systems while eliminating excess fat and cellulite and building a strong musculature underneath. We are going to examine vitamins, minerals and extracts that strengthen and repair these vital systems. The substances listed below can be taken in the form of vitamin supplements or as "superfoods." All are healthy, natural and you may already consume many of them on a daily basis. Many of them also are available as topical solutions.

Some natural food proponents claim it's more effective to ingest vitamins as food rather than in pill form. Our bodies may absorb them more readily from food than from supplements–but it's more important to *get them in you* than to be overly concerned about what form they go in as.

Below is a comprehensive index of vitamins, minerals, supplements and other substances that support and enhance skin, lymphatics and connective tissue. Consuming as many of them as you reasonably can on a daily basis will give your body the fuel it needs to do its job. As with anything, please consult your health care provider before making changes to your diet.

You can buy many of the substances listed below as individual topical ingredients that you can combine to make your own customized skin-firming treatments. This is a great way to have better control over the substances you're putting on your body and to reduce associated costs. In most cases, when you make your own at-home solutions, you'll want to use the freshest ingredients possible and keep them refrigerated between uses to help them stay fresh and effective.

Maximum benefits will come from 1) consuming these effective substances either as healthy superfoods or as supplements and 2) using these effective substances as external lotions *at the same time*. This two-pronged approach will ensure our skin gets the repairing substances it needs via two effective methods–internally and externally. I have noted which agents are appropriate to take internally, which are external only, and which are both. The most effective use when a substance can be taken internally or externally may be to do both–consume it, and use it as a lotion–as long as your doctor agrees.

To save you time and effort in trying to hunt these various substances down, visit this book's website at www.firmlooseskin.com where you will find links to all these substances on Amazon.com. You can also shop for these skin-firming substances directly on Amazon at http://astore.amazon.com/firlooski-20. The Amazon tie-in site is organized by substance, making it easy to find the supplements and extracts detailed below.

You also can visit your local grocery store or pharmacy, specialty supplement store (like GNC) or search the Internet for the very best prices and highest quality on these. If you order online, be sure to factor shipping into the total price you pay. The prices listed below are not meant to be comprehensive but are suggestive of what is available as of fall 2012, and I strongly encourage you to shop around to compare price and quality before purchasing since price and availability of anything varies from minute to minute on the Internet, as you know.

When shopping for supplements and external treatments, measurements, unfortunately, aren't standardized. You may see g (grams), mg (milligrams), mcg (micrograms), IU (international units) or other units of measurement. Always take note of the amount you should be taking and the amount the substance you're purchasing has.

If you need to convert measurement units from grams to milligrams to micrograms to international units, a quick Internet search for "mg to mcg" or "IU to mg," etc., will take you to a conversion calculator. If the RDA of a substance is 55 mcg you don't want to confuse that with 55 mg or you may be wasting money on a product that's far stronger than you need, or even putting yourself at risk for overdose. 1 g = 1,000 mg = 1,000,000 mcg; IUs vary from substance to substance and should be searched individually.

When purchasing these supplements and substances, compare the RDA or other suggested amount with the actual active ingredient percentages in what you ultimately buy. If the RDA is, for example, 300 mg, and the tablets you buy are 600 mg, you can use a pill cutter to halve the tablets, saving you a lot of money.

Unfortunately, you can't split capsules or gelcaps without making a big mess–don't try. Instead try to find purchases as close to the RDA as possible. For example, if the RDA is 400 mg there's no need to take 1000 mg capsules instead, and so on.

RDA as a measurement is more important for supplements you take internally than for external treatments since possible overdose risks for external supplements tend to be lower. Unnecessarily high concentrations of substances may be irritating to the skin, however, so exercise caution, use common sense and clear it with your doctor before you incorporate any of these items into your daily routine.

Hundreds of lotions are marketed to consumers for tightening skin, but are any of them effective? A lot is going to depend on what the lotion or crème targets and what it contains.

As we have learned, building and repairing collage and elastin is the key to tightening skin since loose skin needs to rebond to the underlying muscle through connective tissue. Strengthening our connective tissue, primarily through supporting the repair and production of collagen and through supporting the health of our lymph systems, is a key way to firm our skin.

Be wary, suspicious and discerning when selecting external treatments to help repair your skin. Topical treatments that don't target the right things simply aren't going to be effective. That being said, it's certainly not impossible for a lotion or other treatment to help. In fact, dozens of scientific studies show that collagen repair is possible and that some external treatments are effective.

In making a determination on which substances or treatments to purchase, we will want to examine each using the following criteria:

- ingredients
- amount/percentage of active ingredients
- claims
- testimonials
- guarantees

You will notice I have not factored in cost as a criterion. This is because, to me, cost does not matter. This is not because I have a money tree growing in my yard! I look at it this way: it doesn't matter how inexpensive a lotion that claims to firm skin is; if it doesn't work, I'm not going to buy it. On the other hand, if a lotion comes along that has ingredients I know make sense, in amounts that make sense, with enough real testimonials to its effectiveness, and that has an iron-clad money-back guarantee, then frankly, cost isn't going to be the deciding factor, because I'm not going to choose a less expensive and less effective substitute, nor should you. That truly would be a waste of money.

Try to avoid external crèmes or lotions that contain alcohol and fragrance. These ingredients won't help firm your skin and may cause you unnecessary sensitivity. This may mean you'll need to mix and create your own customized crèmes and lotions—which in the long run may prove much less costly and far more effective. Where available, oils, extracts and serums will probably be a better choice because they will have fewer extraneous ingredients that we simply don't need to use or to pay extra for.

To be truly effective, presumably a lotion should include as many of these ingredients as possible. Since no crème or lotion contains every single ingredient mentioned below, using a variety of external preparations, or, better yet, combining individual ingredients to make our own custom preparations, seems to make the most sense.

To avoid possible interactions, it would be best to use different topical treatments on a varying schedule of your choosing—every other day, morning/evening, and so on. And, as with internally taken supplements, check with your doctor before using any of these, and be sure to test each on an inconspicuous area of your body, such as the inner fold of your elbow, before slathering them on. Your face is your billboard—***never*** put ***anything*** on your face before you've tested it somewhere else on your body. Any substance listed below may be used externally; however, I wouldn't recommend taking any of the external-only substances listed below internally.

I also would not recommend going out and buying every single supplement on this list and taking them all for the first time at once, particularly if you are not in the habit of taking a daily multivitamin. Incorporate them one or a few at the time to give your body time to adjust as needed and as your doctor advises.

Again, you can visit the website, www.firmlooseskin.com, which links to a frequently updated list of all of these substances on Amazon.com to make them easy to find. Since a book can't stay as updated as a website, visit the website or shop Amazon directly at http://astore.amazon.com/firlooski-20.

Below is the list of skin-firming substances that seem to provide the best results in helping to repair connective tissue through building collagen and elastin, reduce cellulite, support healthy lymph functioning and/or improve skin. Several easy-to-use resources are included at the end of this chapter. First is a list of substances by which skin-firming approach they target: collagen growth, connective tissue repair, lymphatic repair, cellulite reduction, skin repair and muscle repair, to help you assess which areas you need the most support for.

Next is a table of recommended daily allowances of each substance listed below. Note that typical recommended daily allowances are based on adults over the age of 18 and by gender, where applicable. Typically, these substances do not come with recommended dosages specific to firming loose skin–however, ensuring that you are getting the recommended daily allowance of each should be a good start. Use this list when researching which substances to purchase.

Following that is a list of internal substances, alphabetically, then external substances, alphabetically, and finally a list of superfoods by food group and some of the vitamins and minerals each contains. These lists can easily be reproduced and will be useful when shopping for or discussing these substances with your health care provider.

It's worth mentioning again–none of the information in this book constitutes medical advice and it should not be treated as such. Get your doctor's permission before you add any new substances to your diet or put any new substances on your skin. Some substances may cause side effects, which are noted in abbreviated form in the table at the end of this section. Some substances may interact with medications which is another reason to check with your doctor before taking anything new. Most importantly, do not use any of these supplements or external treatments (or any supplement or treatment!) if you are pregnant or nursing unless your doctor specifically tells you to.

Skin-Tightening Substances, Vitamin A to Zinc

External and Internal: **Vitamin A** as **Beta-Carotene** is an antioxidant that gives certain vegetables and fruits a distinct orange or red color. It promotes connective tissue growth and repair. It may also have a positive effect on sun-damaged skin. Beta-carotene is a very safe supplement. The U.S. government reports that ingesting large amounts of beta-carotene generally is not dangerous. The RDA (recommended daily allowance) of vitamin A is 900 mcg for men and 700 mcg for women. Beta-carotene supplements start at around $3 per 100 for 25,000 IU which converts to 7,500 mcg–6,600 mcg more than is needed, possibly overkill. A daily multivitamin tablet should have more than enough vitamin A for you to get your RDA and then some.

Vitamin A as **Retinol** may be even more effective as a topical treatment in crèmes and lotions than as an internal supplement. Vitamin A helps our bodies produce collagen according to scientific studies conducted by the U.S. government and a major university. Retinol is a key component of many skin care products. It has been proven to improve skin tone, texture and color, lines and wrinkles and hydration levels.

Note that retinol can cause skin irritation so use sparingly at first, or use gentler solutions before stepping up to stronger ones to build up your tolerance to it. Retinol is available as crèmes and serums and prices vary from under $2 per ounce to over $50 per ounce.

Many foods that contain vitamin A are very healthful and should contribute to your overall skin health. It's best to incorporate both an oral form and a topical form of vitamin A into your skin-firming regimen. Healthy foods that contain vitamin A include:

- cantaloupe
- carrots

- collard greens
- egg yolks
- kale
- low-fat dairy products
- mangoes
- milk
- palm oil
- papayas
- peaches
- pomegranates
- pumpkin
- spinach
- sweet potatoes

External and Internal: **Aescin** is extract of horse chestnut and it has been shown in clinical scientific studies to successfully treat chronic venous insufficiency among other things. It also is used topically for clearing skin conditions. Aescin can improve the condition of our lymph systems since it has been proven in clinical studies to ameliorate post-operative swelling in surgery involving lymph nodes and large limbs.

Aescin may have negative interactions with anticoagulant medication and should not be used if you are prone to edema (swelling). Potential side effects may include gastrointestinal problems (mainly at high doses), dizziness, headaches and itchiness. There is no RDA for aescin but 400-650 mcg should be a fairly effective dose. It may also be used externally as Horse Chestnut Seed Extract which typically contains 2% aescin and it generally is applied 3-4 times daily. In capsule form, typical prices start at under $10 for 90 capsules and under $15 for four ounces of the crème product.

External: Who hasn't experienced the pain of a sunburn? **Aloe Vera** is a wonderful substance that reduces the pain, swelling, dryness and flaking that comes from a nasty sunburn. It's also antimicrobial, antibacterial and antifungal. Best of all, it helps stimulate collagen production—and it's very inexpensive at less than $10 for 13+ ounces. Aloe vera definitely should be in your arsenal of skin-firming treatments.

External: **Alpha-Hydroxy Acids** (there are more than one) refer to several types of external treatments which are becoming increasingly popular as skin-care ingredients. They are anti-inflammatory and exfoliating, and in concentrated form, they are used as chemical peels under a doctor's supervision. They may not directly contribute to firming skin but use of them should approve the appearance of your outer skin.

I wouldn't recommend them as a primary skin-firming treatment but they can be useful as part of your overall skin regimen. Note that they can be very irritating to the skin and they may cause additional sun sensitivity, so use with caution. Start out using a less-concentrated solution then work your way up to a stronger solution (like an 85% solution), or consider using less irritating **Beta-Hydroxy Acids**, particularly if you already have sensitive skin, detailed below. Prices on this product vary widely, from less than $10 for 7+ ounces to over $15 an ounce for light at-home peels.

Internal: **Alpha Lipoic Acids** are promoted as an anti-aging solution. They are very strong antioxidants that work to repair damaged skin while preventing future skin damage. They are soluble both in oil and water, helping them permeate all parts of a cell. This gives them a very strong ability to fight free radical damage. This antioxidant also boosts vitamin C levels—it's a good weapon to add to our skin-firming arsenal. 200 mg should be an effective amount and this supplement may lower blood sugar so avoid them if you have blood sugar issues. These are a bit more expensive, starting at over $18 for 120 300 mg tablets and up.

Internal: **Amino Acids** are proteins that serve as the building blocks of our bodies, including our muscles, glands, organs, hair and skin, among other things, and they boost the growth and production of connective tissue while helping skin stay hydrated. Key amino acids include **Alanine, Creatine, L-Carnitine, Lysine** and **L-Arginine**, and **L-Ornithine**. Each amino acid has its own specialized function and virtually all of them are important for us in firming our skin. Some help heal, repair and grow muscle tissue; others (like lysine plus L-arginine, for example) help form collagen, others help prevent skin disorders, and still others reduce the appearance of aging. Many have an additional benefit of helping aid weight loss and of increasing energy and metabolism.

An effective dosage for alanine is in the 200-600 mg range and creatine in the 10 g range. Do not exceed this since high doses may cause liver or kidney damage. Consider L-carnitine in the 1-3 g range, lysine + L-arginine in the 1000 mg range and L-ornithine in the 500 mg range (take L-ornithine at bedtime). Do not exceed these since high doses may cause gallstones, impair thyroid, increase blood pressure, impair blood clotting, upset the stomach and/or decrease appetite.

It's easy to find these amino acids sold in combination so take that into consideration when shopping so you don't accidentally purchase the same substance twice.

Combining these amino acids into our diet either as superfoods or as supplements will help our skin, muscles and connective tissue–and as an added benefit, also can help our skin and nails. Amino acids act like skin care from within. Amino acids are a bit on the higher end of pricing, starting at just under $20 for 120 capsules and rising from there.

Amino acids can be taken in supplement form and as superfoods. In particular, eating from these different sources of amino acids helps ensure balance among them. Amino acids are found in these foods:

- beans
- catfish
- cereal grains
- cheese
- chicken
- chickpeas
- cod
- eggs

- fish
- ground beef
- kidney beans
- lamb
- leafy greens
- lentils
- meats
- milk
- navy beans
- nuts
- Parmesan cheese
- pork
- quinoa
- sardines
- soy

Internal: **Antioxidants** prevent molecules in our bodies from oxidizing which can produce free radicals and cause cellular damage. They have been widely studied for their potential to prevent and treat diseases such as cancer and heart disease, among others. Discussed and priced out separately, vitamins C as ascorbic acid and vitamin E are antioxidants. Antioxidants can have a positive effect on the overall condition of our skin and our health in general. The following foods are high in antioxidants:

- beets
- black currants
- blackberries
- blueberries
- concord grapes
- eggplant
- green tea
- plums
- purple cabbage

- purple figs

External and Internal: **Apple Cider Vinegar** makes strong claims to reducing the existence of and improving the external appearance of cellulite and to assisting with weight loss when taken internally. Personally, I love apple cider vinegar because it's a main ingredient in the delicious barbeque sauce native to my home state, Alabama–it's definitely not recommended in *that* form for weight loss, however.

Apple cider vinegar is available at your local grocery store and it's very inexpensive. It's recommended above other types of vinegar like white vinegar for cellulite reduction and weight loss because the process that creates it does not strip it of essential minerals. Used externally, vinegar promotes blood circulation in the skin. It's antiseptic, preventing the growth of bacteria, and it regulates skin pH. Apple cider vinegar can be drunk (generally a couple of tablespoons in a glass of water) but I don't necessarily recommend it–yuck. Consider capsule form instead.

Typical prices start at just over $6 for 240 200 mg capsules. Allergic reactions are rare but may be severe–use caution if you're prone to allergies. You can also mix apple cider vinegar with your favorite crème or oil, like grape seed oil, and apply directly to cellulite-bearing areas.

Don't overdo it as it can irritate skin if overused. You may want to experiment with this. Generally a 50-to-75% mixture should be most effective–three parts vinegar, one part oil, reduce the vinegar concentration if your skin becomes irritated. Refrigerate any unused portion. It could be used on your tossed salad . . . but you can probably find tastier ingredients than these.

Internal: The **B Vitamins** are safe, inexpensive and important both to the lymph system and to connective tissue. **Vitamin B-2**, or riboflavin, is essential to the creation, growth and repair of cells and of connective tissue. Low levels of vitamin B-2 are associated with lymphatic abnormalities. The RDA of vitamin B-2 is 1.3 mg for men and 1.1 mg for women; taking excessive amounts of B-2 daily (over 10 mg) can increase eye sensitivity to sunlight and can contribute to eye damage if you don't wear sunglasses outdoors, so don't overdo it. Vitamin B-2 is found in the following foods:

- avocados
- broccoli
- cheese
- currants
- dark green leafy vegetables
- eggs
- milk
- nuts
- oily fish
- organ meats
- yeast

Vitamin B-3, also known as niacin, is used to treat circulatory problems and a vitamin B-3 deficiency can lead to skin that is sensitive to light, thick, rough, dry and prone to outbreaks and eruptions. The RDA for vitamin B-3 is 16 mg for men and 14 mg for women; taking amounts in excess of 50 mg per day can cause skin heat flushes, liver damage and stomach ulcers so don't overdo it. Foods that contain vitamin B-3 include:

- beef
- pork
- fish
- milk
- cheese
- whole wheat
- potatoes
- corn
- carrots

Vitamin B-6, also known as pyridoxine, has been shown to improve lymphatic drainage which is important for carrying toxins away from the skin and throughout the entire body. It is involved in metabolizing fats and carbohydrates and it promotes healthy skin. The RDA of B-6 is 1.3 mg for men or women. Taking excessive amounts of B-6 (over 100 mg per day) can cause serious nerve damage so definitely don't overdo it with this one either. Vitamin B-6 is found in:

- chicken
- fish
- pork
- eggs
- milk
- liver
- wheat germ
- kidneys
- brewer's yeast

B-Complex vitamins combine all three and are very inexpensive, starting at just over $14 for 360 tablets, or you can purchase the B-vitamins separately as well.

External: **Beta-Hydroxy Acid/Salicylic Acid** has been studied for its effect on prematurely aged, over-tanned skin. It exfoliates and improves skin color and texture and it's also an effective acne treatment. Some studies show that salicylic acid works similarly to alpha-hydroxy acid but is less irritating. Both alpha- and beta-hydroxy acid can cause skin irritation, redness and dryness so use intelligently and stop using if you have an adverse reaction. With either, start out with a less-intensive solution and work your way up to a stronger solution, like a 30% solution, over time.

Using a product with alpha- or beta-hydroxy acid should help your overall skin appearance. Beta-hydroxy acid ranges in price from $25 for 8+ ounces to $20+ per ounce for light at-home peels.

Internal: **Bioflavonoids** are produced by plants and they are found in many foods rich in vitamin C. Bioflavonoids give plants yellow, red and blue coloration. In connective tissue, they can repair damage by increasing the synthesis of collagen. They improve the absorption of vitamin C and, to be most effective, both should be taken together.

There is no RDA for bioflavenoids but amounts under 250 mg generally are thought to be safe. Amounts over 250 mg may elevate estrogen levels or cause allergic reactions so use cautiously. Bioflavonoids are very inexpensive, starting at just over $6 for 100 tables, and are found in these foods:

- apricots
- black currants
- buckwheat
- cherries
- chervil
- citrus fruits
- elderberries
- grapefruit
- grapes
- hawthorn berry
- horsetail
- peppers
- prunes
- rosehips

External and Internal: **Vitamin C** as **Ascorbic Acid**, its purest form, is involved in hundreds of vital processes within the body and it promotes the development of strong connective tissue. It forms collagen and new blood vessels and it slows the erosion of cartilage. It can help reduce the swelling of connective tissue as well as joint and muscle pain and stiffness. Vitamin C eliminates free radicals, the highly charged oxygen molecules mentioned in section one, caused by ultraviolet rays. Vitamin C is the only antioxidant that stimulates the synthesis of collagen. Studies have shown that vitamin C minimizes lines and wrinkles.

Vitamin C as **L-Ascorbic Acid** should be used externally. It is available as a crème or serum and prices vary widely–from just under $8 for 1.8 ounces to over $30 an ounce in serum form. Work your way up slowly to a 25% percent solution, the most effective dose, to avoid skin irritation.

Internal vitamin C deficiency can keep wounds from healing. In fact, extreme vitamin C deficiency causes scurvy, a painful connective tissue disease which causes tooth loss, skin discoloration and makes wounds much harder to heal. Scurvy was fairly common two centuries ago among sailors at sea and others deprived of vitamin C-containing foods. Vitamin C truly is crucial to a healthy body, a healthy immune system and healthy connective tissue.

The RDA of vitamin C is 90 mg for men and 75 mg for women but it's easy to find C supplements with dosages in the thousands of mg. Side effects at high doses are mild and generally include stomach upset. At a minimum, get your RDA of vitamin C; this is one supplement where the more, the merrier, as long as your physician agrees. C is easily found in daily multivitamins and that's probably the most cost-effective way to get your daily vitamin C. Also sold separately, vitamin C supplements are relatively inexpensive, starting at around $9 for 150 tablets. Foods high in vitamin C include:

- bell peppers
- broccoli
- Brussels sprouts
- Goji berries
- kiwi
- leafy greens, particularly kale and spinach
- oranges and citrus fruits
- papaya
- pomegranates
- watermelon

External: **Caffeine**, used externally as a lotion or crème (but not as your favorite mocha skim latte, unfortunately) provides multiple skin-tightening benefits. External caffeine reduces excess fluids by dehydrating skin. Some believe it can burn fat in the skin and that it can effectively target cellulite with its fluid-reducing properties.

Caffeine also is a strong antioxidant which scavenges free radicals and it may help protect our skin against ultraviolet rays. Caffeine crème can help tighten the skin by encouraging the production of elastin and collagen. Prices vary widely and start at around $4 for 2 ounces; a 5% solution should be effective. You can also make your own by adding fresh, caffeinated, unused coffee grounds to your favorite crème or lotion. Mix approximately one-third part fresh coffee grounds to two-thirds lotion, like a vitamin E crème or grape seed oil, for example, and massage thoroughly into skin. Leave on for 10-15 minutes then rinse off. Keep mixture refrigerated for freshness.

External and Internal: **Calcium**, a mineral, is well known as a building block for healthy bones and teeth but it also positively impacts muscle growth and overall health. Calcium also helps maintain cell permeability. Calcium is rare to find as a single ingredient in a lotion but often is combined with other age-fighting ingredients.

The RDA of calcium is 1000 mg for men and women both; high doses may cause constipation, stomach upset, irregular heartbeat and kidney damage so don't overdo it. Calcium supplement prices vary widely, starting at around $10 for 100 500 mg capsules. Foods high in calcium include:

- almonds
- argula
- beans
- blackstrap molasses
- broccoli
- chia seeds

- dairy products
- dark leafy greens
- dried fruits and nuts
- dried herbs
- flax seeds
- kale
- oatmeal
- oranges
- quinoa
- salmon
- sesame seeds
- soy milk
- sunflower seeds
- tofu

External: **Cocoa Butter** has long been used to prevent and reduce the appearance of stretch marks and some claim it can reduce the appearance of cellulite as well. It is a natural antioxidant and it has definite skin-smoothing and skin-moisturizing properties. Look for 100% cocoa butter with no additives. Cocoa butter is inexpensive with prices starting at around $5 for 7 ounces.

External and Internal: **Co-enzyme Q10** as **Ubiquinol** is an antioxidant and it provides energy to cells. It can assist in the production of collagen and elastin. It has an added benefit of helping to aid weight loss by improving the energy levels in cells, contributing to a faster metabolism. Incorporating co-enzyme Q10 into your diet can help you lose weight. It works well as a supplement and a lotion.

Ubiquinol lotions tend to feature other age-fighting ingredients; capsules are fairly expensive, starting at just over $40 for 120 100 mg. Non-ubiquinol COQ10 capsules are much less expensive, starting at just over $13 for the same count. The RDA of COQ10 is 30-200 mg for men and women. High doses may upset your stomach and/or lower blood sugar so avoid COQ10 if you have blood sugar issues.

Foods that contain co-enzyme Q10 include:

- beef liver
- broccoli
- canola oil
- chicken
- mackerel
- nuts
- parsley
- pork
- soybeans
- yellowtail tuna

External: **Collagen Supplements** like **DHEA** (dehydroepiandrosterone, a steroid hormone produced by our adrenal glands) are controversial as skin firming ingredients. Claims exist that hydrolyzed collagen supplements can restore collagen and reverse the aging process. Many products marketed as collagen supplements or collagen-based beauty products contain hydrolyzed collagen. However, there is a lack of evidence that collagen supplements can benefit your skin. Further, DHEA treatments may cause hormonal side effects, particularly in men. In this book, we are concentrating on effective treatments that help your body rebuild and strengthen its own collagen so, until DHEA and other collagen supplements come with more substantive proof, let's skip them in favor of other treatments with a better track record.

External: **Copper** is a trace mineral that produces hemoglobin in red blood cells. Copper may also improve the strength of connective tissue. It enhances production of collagen for connective tissue repair. Copper also works with vitamin C to produce elastin. Note that consuming too much copper can cause diarrhea, cramps, nausea and can lead to problems like depression, insomnia and even more serious mental and physical problems, so it's best not to incorporate a strong copper supplement into your diet but to concentrate on external applications and superfoods with trace amounts of copper instead.

Copper peptides are an antioxidant and they support our body in producing elastin and collagen. Copper peptides also remove damaged elastin and collagen from scar tissue. Side effects generally are mild but may include redness, burning, rashes and skin inflammation. If you experience any of this discontinue use.

This is definitely a substance we want to add to our skin-firming arsenal. Look for a solution with .1% copper peptides or more. Prices start at around $35 an ounce. Foods that contain trace amounts of copper include:

- almonds
- beans
- calamari
- crab
- dried herbs
- hazelnuts
- liver
- lobster
- nuts
- oysters
- pistachios
- roasted pumpkin seeds
- roasted squash seeds
- sesame seeds
- shellfish
- soybeans
- sun dried tomatoes
- sunflower seeds
- tahini
- tomatoes

- unsweetened cocoa powder

External and Internal: **Vitamin E** is an antioxidant that slows bodily oxidation due to free radicals and promotes skin health and longevity. It is important to protecting and maintaining cell membranes, promoting the healing of injured tissues and it is believed to reduce scarring from injuries. Vitamin E is critical to healthy skin. It protects the epidermis and contributes to repairing connective tissue. Vitamin E is used to increase skin health as a food, a vitamin supplement, and as an external crème.

Vitamin E crème can be found very inexpensively, with prices starting at less than $4 for 4 ounces. Capsules are also inexpensive, starting at just over $12 for 500 of 400 IU. The RDA of vitamin E is 15 mg (22.4 IU–E is commonly dosed in IU) for men and women. High doses may thin blood and E may interact with medications so check with your doctor to avoid possible drug interactions.

This is another vitamin it's probably more cost-effective to take as part of a multivitamin if possible. Vitamin E is found in these foods:

- almonds and other nuts
- asparagus
- avocados
- eggs
- kale
- sunflower and other seeds
- vegetable oils

Internal: **Ellagic Acid** is an antioxidant that fights free radical damage and it has been promoted as a natural cancer-fighting method. It actively prevents the destruction of collagen and swelling caused by exposure to ultraviolet radiation and it is a promising treatment for wrinkles caused by tanning.

Be sure not to take an ellagic acid supplement made from raspberry leaves if you are pregnant as it may cause premature labor. High doses may increase blood pressure so avoid this substance if that's a problem for you. There is no RDA for ellagic acid but 40-900 mg should be a fairly effective dose. Supplement prices start at just under $7 for 60 500 mg tablets. Foods that contain ellagic acid (dried berries are a primary source) include:

- apples
- blackberries
- blueberries
- cherries
- cranberries
- grapes
- peaches
- pecans
- pomegranates
- red raspberries
- strawberries
- walnuts

External: **Essential Oils**, made from plant sources like flowers and fruit, have long been used as components of aromatherapy to provide physical, emotional, beauty and other benefits. Some essential oils are promoted as having cellulite-reducing and skin-improving benefits. **Grape Seed Oil** and **Grape Seed Extract** are produced by pressing the essential oil from the seeds of grapes. Grape seed oil is sold as a fine cooking oil and food grade oil is best for skin firming uses–plus, it's very inexpensive.

Mustard Oil also can firm, restore elasticity to, and reduce the signs of aging in skin.

Essential oils are very strong so they should be mixed with other substances before skin application, such as mixing mustard oil with grape seed oil. You can heat an essential oil mixture before or after applying it to the skin to help it soak in (with warm compresses or a heating pad). I have traded in my expensive night crème for simple grape seed oil and the results so far are better while costing 95% less. An excellent trade!

Various other essential oils which may be helpful to the skin include basil, cedarwood, clary, cypress, fennel, juniper, lemon, orange, patchouli, rosemary, sage and thyme. Any of these essential oils can be mixed with grape seed oil–using no more than five-to-ten drops each to a few ounces of a base oil like grape seed or coconut oil–to make a pleasant-smelling solution that may help your skin.

Essential oils as a skin-firming treatment may work, or they may not. Traditional science hasn't studied the effects of essential oils to improving skin to the same extent vitamins and minerals have been studied, so they likely are best as a less-important part of your overall skin-firming routine. Basically, use them if you like them but don't feel like you need to or have to in order to get the same results we hope to get from other substances.

Prices on essential oils vary widely but in general they are fairly inexpensive. Grape seed oil may be a purchase you decide to make the next time you're at the grocery store–the oil you cook with is the same oil you can use on your skin. It can also be found online for around $3 for 4 ounces. Grape seed extract is a bit more pricey, starting at just over $16 for 90 250 mg capsules, and 50-100 mg should be a fairly effective dose. Mustard oil starts at just under $10 for 500 ml–also a bit pricey but not prohibitively so.

Internal: **Glucosamine** is an antioxidant and a component of the connective tissue and of ligaments and tendons. It is involved in preserving joint structure and it frequently is used to treat arthritis and joint problems. When applied topically, glucosamine stimulates cell renewal through rehydration, replacing old, wrinkled skin with fresh, healthy skin and stimulating the production of collagen through the production of hyaluronic acid, which rebuilds skin tissue. Find glucosamine crème as a component of methylsulfonylmethane (MSM) lotion, detailed below as a separate substance.

Note that some glucosamine supplements are made from shellfish so if you are allergic to shellfish, be sure to use supplements derived from other sources. Also, some glucosamine supplements include chondroitin, which seems to have little benefit to rebuilding connective tissue, so taking glucosamine/chondroitin supplements would be unnecessary to help firm skin, although they certainly have other benefits. Glucosamine may cause stomach upset and diarrhea. It also may raise blood pressure and cholesterol levels so avoid it if you have these concerns.

Glucosamine naturally occurs in the cartilage and shells of shellfish but not in the meat, so taking a supplement or applying a topical solution is necessary. Prices for glucosamine start at around $12.50 for 150 1500 mg tablets, which happens to be the RDA for this supplement. You can also find glucosamine tablets coupled with methylsulfonylmethane (MSM) which is discussed below.

Internal: **Gotu Kola** is an herb commonly used in traditional Chinese medicine to treat bacterial, viral and parasitic infections, fatigue, various emotional disorders including anxiety and depression, to improve memory and intelligence, and for wound healing and circulation problems. Certain chemicals found in gotu kola seem to decrease swelling and blood pressure in veins and, most importantly for us, increase collagen production. Ingesting large quantities of gotu kola may cause headaches, liver damage, skin allergies, stomach upset, drowsiness and it may interfere with hypoglycemic medication. Do not use gotu kola if you have or are at risk for skin cancer.

Common methods of taking gotu kola include as a supplement in pill form or as a tea. The most commonly recommended supplement to take is listed as gotu kola, hydrocotyle asiaticam extract of Indian pennywort with 70% triterpenic acids. Gotu kola can easily be found on the Internet, including from Amazon.com, and it may be available from your local pharmacy or health food store. Prices vary; supplements start at just under $6 for 1 ounce as a liquid supplement and just over $6 for 100 475 mg capsules. The standard dosage, analogous to RDA, of gotu kola is 1000-4000 mg daily. For safety's sake, be sure you know the country of origin of this and any other supplement you buy.

External and Internal: **Green Tea** and **Green Tea Extract** are high in antioxidants and help firm skin both as a healthy drink that also promotes weight loss, and as a supplement. Green tea helps protect the skin from free radical damage and contains **Methylxanthines** (so does caffeine) that increase skin circulation. Methylxanthines are used as an effective treatment for cellulite. Green tea reduces skin swelling and has a positive effect on collagen production. It also protects against skin damage when applied externally.

In addition to drinking green tea, you can apply green tea directly to your skin by dampening a tea bag and holding it to your skin, or you can buy it as a crème or lotion. Prices start at around $13 for 8 ounces of lotion.

You can buy regular green tea to drink at your local grocery store; in capsule form, green tea extract starts at around $14 for 180 500 mg capsules. The standard dosage, analogous to RDA, is 100-750 mg per day. As with any substance containing caffeine, it may cause irritability, insomnia, heart palpitations and dizziness if consumed in large quantities so use common sense if adding green tea or green tea extract to your diet—check the caffeine content.

External: **Hyaluronic Acid,** also known as a glycosaminoglycan, often is used in conjunction with vitamin C and it has been advertised as a substance that can reverse aging through treating wrinkles. It is a component of connective tissue and a lubricant and it has excellent reviews as a potential skin-firming substance. Capsules start at around $16 for 60 100 mg capsules; two ounces of serum starts at around $15. Look for 100% hyaluronic acid in preparations you buy. Side effects generally are mild and may include slight skin reactions.

External: **Kinetin** promotes cell division and it encourages the production of collagen in the skin. It may also act as an antioxidant when it comes into contact with the skin. It has not been proven as being as effective as retinol, green tea or vitamin E but it may be a bit less irritating than retinol, so it's a good secondary ingredient to consider.

Prices vary widely on kinetin but less-expensive versions start at around $14 for half an ounce. Favor preparations containing .03% to .1% solutions. Side effects generally are rare but may include allergic reactions. Avoid kinetin if you're prone to serious allergies.

External and Internal: **Lycopene** is a pigment found in fruits and vegetables giving them red, orange or yellow pigmentation that can reduce free radicals, create stronger cell junctions, protect against ultraviolet damage and reduce facial redness, among other things. Important to firming our skin, lycopene can tighten cell junctions which bind cells together and provide a barrier to help the cell decide what gets inside it and what doesn't. This helps cells retain moisture.

Note that overconsumption of lycopene can cause stomach upset and it also may cause a temporary yellow or orange tint to your skin, so don't overdo it, and if you do, simply cut back on lycopene until your skin color normalizes. This is not a reason to avoid lycopene, however. Lycopene crème starts at over $25 per ounce; supplements are a bit less costly, starting at around $9 for 60 25 mg tablets. The RDA for lycopene is 10-30 mg per day for men and women. Foods that contain lycopene include:

- apricots
- guava
- papayas
- pink grapefruit
- red bell peppers
- red carrots
- rosehips
- tomatoes
- watermelon

Internal: **Manganese** supports bone growth and repair, it enables the body to utilize the B and C vitamins and it acts as an antioxidant. Manganese contributes to building collagen and it is active in DNA repair. Note that small amounts of manganese are plenty and overdoses can be very dangerous, causing nervous system damage and a host of other problems including hallucinations–don't overdo it. Most individual manganese supplements seem to contain far more than you're going to want to take unless your doctor specifically directs you too.

The RDA of manganese is small–2.3 mg for men and 1.8 for women. Supplements start at just over $7 for 100 10 mg capsules which is a lot so look for a multivitamin with a lower dose instead, look for tablets you can split with a pill splitter, or just rely on these superfoods for the manganese you need:

- almonds
- avocados
- brown rice
- coffee
- eggs
- leafy greens
- liver
- spices
- tea
- walnuts
- whole grains

External and Internal: **Methylsulfonylmethane** (MSM) contains sulfur and it is helpful for many body functions. It is primarily used to treat arthritis and muscle pain, and it can help build collagen. Methylsulfonylmethane can reverse hair loss and some report that it helps tighten loose skin. MSM can be used orally or topically. Capsules start at just over $14 for 240 1000 mg; lotion pricing starts at around $17 for 16 ounces. An effective amount of MSM should be in the 2-6 g range. Serious allergic reactions are possible but rare. Side effects may include nausea, diarrhea, headache and fatigue. Foods containing MSM include:

- chives
- cow's milk
- garlic
- leeks
- onions
- shallots

Internal: **Omega 3 Fatty Acids** like **Fish Oil** are supplements that benefit our skin. Fish oil helps skin maintain elasticity and firmness, helps us avoid wrinkles, and it helps balance out the moisture content of our cells. It has been used to treat skin conditions like eczema, psoriasis, acne and rashes, among other things, and a lack of omega 3 fatty acid can contribute to dandruff and dry flaky skin. Be sure to get a fish oil supplement ***with*** EPA (eicosapentaenoic acid) and ***without*** DHA (docosahexaenoic acid) which isn't necessary for skin care. The RDA of fish oil is 180 mg for men or women. Side effects may include bloating, gas, diarrhea and it may thin your blood.

Prices for EPA fish oil start at a fraction over $25 for 400 1000 mg capsules. Foods high in omega 3s include:

- broccoli
- fish oil
- flax seeds or flax seed oil
- green leafy vegetables
- hemp
- salmon
- spinach
- walnuts

Internal: **Protein** is necessary to support every system in your body and it is necessary to build strong connective tissue. Protein supports the functioning of every other potential treatment listed in this section. Protein supplements typically will be unnecessary. Foods high in protein include:

- chicken
- cod
- crab
- eggs
- lobster
- seaweed

External and Internal: **Punicalagin** and **Quercetin** are antioxidants with anti-inflammatory properties. Punicalagin helps to protect cartilage, a connective tissue. Quercetin helps diminish free radicals at the site of inflammation.

Quercetin is found in tea; supplements start in the $12 range for 100 500 mg capsules. 200-500 mg should be a fairly effective dose; more than 1 g may damage kidneys so don't overdo it.

Punicalagin is found in lotions with prices starting in the $22 for 4 ounces range. Punicalagin also is found in the following foods:

- pomegranates
- red raspberries

External and Internal: **Resveratrol** is an emollient, lubricant, antioxidant and anti-inflammatory that fights aging. Resveratrol capsules start at under $24 for 120 200 mg (a fairly effective dose should range from around 100 to 500 mg); crème starts at just over $11 for 6 ounces. Do not take resveratrol if you have had or are at risk for breast cancer. Grape seed extract, discussed above, is an excellent source of resveratrol, as are these foods:

- cinnamon
- coffee
- olive oil
- oregano
- soy
- tea

External and Internal: **Seabuckthorn** is a plant that is an antioxidant that fights free radical damage, reduces swelling, discourages immune system attacks, is antimicrobial, regulates hormones, and softens scars, among other things. It has been used as a treatment for acne. Seabuckthorn extract can be made from both the berries and the leaves and seems to have the potential to be effective as a topical solution.

For supplements, prices vary widely and start at around $9 for 100 capsules; as a topical solution, seabuckthorn oil starts at less than $9 for 10 ml. There is no RDA for seabuckthorn but 500 mg or 300 ml of extract should be a fairly effective dose. Seabuckthorn may interact with other medications so, as with anything, check with your doctor before you start taking it.

External and Internal: **Seaweed**, including **Phytessence Wakame** (Undaria pinnatifida) and **Hijiki** (Hijikia fusiformis), is found naturally in the Sea of Japan. It contains amino acids, antioxidants, a plethora of vitamins and minerals, and glutamic acid, among other things. It also contains a compound called **Fucoxanthin**, which may help with fat loss.

Seaweed is purported to have many health benefits including reducing connective tissue problems and arthritis pain, reducing skin inflammation, protecting against sun exposure and reducing the breakdown of collagen and elastin while supporting the rebuilding of both substances in our skin. Some also claim that it helps reduce cellulite.

It can be used externally on the skin but there's no solid indication that external treatments work best for firming the skin. Probably a better way to get this important substance into your system is going to be internally, either by adding wakame and hijiki to your diet or by taking them as a seaweed extract supplement or fucoxanthin supplement. Seaweed extract isn't cheap and neither is fucoxanthin—both start at over $20 a bottle for 90 capsules—but wakame and hijiki as superfoods are relatively inexpensive, although for some they are an acquired taste and not as potent as seafood extract.

If you choose to try seaweed as a superfood rather than an extract, you should be able to find wakame and hijiki at your local specialty supermarket or Asian grocery store or you can easily order them online.

External and Internal: **Selenium** is a mineral with antioxidant properties that protects skin from sun damage. Selenium also plays a major role in keeping the skin more firm and elastic. Note that selenium should only be consumed in trace amounts.

One inexpensive way to use selenium topically is to buy Selsun Blue dandruff shampoo—it's a key ingredient, just rinse thoroughly, or look for it as an additional ingredient in another lotion you decide to buy.

It's also available as an inexpensive lotion, starting at just over $6 for 75 ml, and as an inexpensive supplement, starting at around $7 for 100 200 mg capsules. Buy a pill splitter and split higher dosage pills if necessary since the RDA for selenium is only 55 mcg for men or women, or, better yet, just look for a multivitamin that contains selenium. High dosages may increase the risk of developing diabetes and skin cancer and may cause other skin reactions so definitely don't overdo it with this one.

Selenium occurs naturally in:

- Brazil nuts
- eggs
- mushrooms
- oysters
- pasta
- shrimp

- sunflower seeds
- turkey

External and Internal: **Silica** is a mineral that helps protect against sun damage. It is found in bones, hair, fingernails and skin, all of which depend on silica for strength and flexibility. Silica is a major component of collagen and the highest concentration of silica in our bodies is found in the connective tissue.

It can be found very inexpensively and commonly as "**Horsetail**" (**Equisetum**, an antioxidant)–at just over $3 for 90 500 mg capsules or just under $9 for 4 ounces of lotion.

The RDA of silica is 900 mg per day for men or women. Do not take silica if you have heart or kidney disease, diabetes or gout. Do not drink alcohol heavily and do not use nicotine patches or nicotine gum and silica at the same time.

Foods that are natural sources of silica include:

- fruit
- whole grains

Internal: **Water!** Water makes up between half and two-thirds of the human body. Women are on the lower end, towards half, men on the higher, closer to two-thirds. Obesity can lower this percentage to less than half. In contrast, infants' bodies may be composed of nearly three-quarters water. Water is crucial to good health.

Do you drink enough water every day? Many diets recommend that, at a minimum–minimum!–you should be drinking eight 8-ounce glasses of water daily, more if you are trying to lose weight or tighten your skin. It's not uncommon for people on diets to drink double this amount–a gallon–or more, daily. Drinking adequate water is necessary for your health, your body, to lose weight, and to improve your complexion as well as the condition of your skin. Drink your water!

Note that I specified water. Not diet drinks or colas, not coffee or tea, not beer or wine, not other flavored beverages—water. You should be drinking your water in addition to any other beverages you drink on a daily basis.

When you don't drink enough water you can become dehydrated. Most of us have experienced dehydration at one time or another, and, as you know, it's unpleasant and uncomfortable. Being dehydrated dries out your skin, and, over time, can cause it to wrinkle, sag and droop. Lines and creases can stand out more. In contrast, hydration will have a positive impact on your skin and more importantly on your connective tissue and lymph system.

In the first section we learned that connective tissue is crucial to tightening skin. One published scientific study examined the influence of hydration on aging connective tissue and found that connective tissue and tendons elongate and are more flexible when enough water is present. This is very important. Hydration improves how flexible your connective tissue is, and the flexibility of your connective tissue is a major factor in getting your loose skin to adhere to the underlying muscle.

Drinking water alone won't firm up all your loose skin if you have a lot, like I do. But <u>not</u> drinking water is not doing your connective tissue any favors. For the sake of your connective tissue, drink your water!

External and Internal: **Zinc** is essential to the production of connective tissue, cartilage and bone, and it has been shown to help arthritis. Zinc is an antioxidant and, along with copper and manganese, it helps neutralize free radical activity and joint inflammation and it stimulates the immune system.

The RDA of zinc is 11 mg for men and 8 mg for women. Zinc supplements are very inexpensive, starting at just over $5 for 120 30 mg tablets and around $10 for 5 ounces of lotion. Excessive amounts may cause flu-like symptoms, anemia, hallucinations and more, and it may raise cholesterol levels, so don't overdo it with zinc. Foods containing zinc include:

- beans
- cheese
- egg whites
- lamb
- lentils
- mushrooms
- oysters
- pumpkin seeds
- sardines
- tofu
- whole grains

Note that, a great way to save money is to take a **daily multivitamin** that incorporates as many of these substances as possible into a single tablet. Keep this in mind when shopping for the substances detailed above.

When considering which of these substances to eat as superfoods, to take as supplements or to use as external lotions, use common sense. If you are allergic to, have a great dislike for, or are on a diet that restricts any of these foods, choose something else.

Check with your doctor before taking any new supplements or using any new crèmes or lotions. Perform a skin patch test, such as in the fold of your elbow, to test for sensitivity or allergy before slathering anything new on your body. Read and follow the directions that come with any substance you purchase. And don't go out and try to incorporate every single substance into your personal skin routine tomorrow.

If you want to concentrate on a few at first then branch out into others, think long and hard about incorporating **retinol, vitamins C** and **E, copper peptides, hyaluronic acid, seaweed extract** and **silica** in first then the others as you go along. All the substances listed above are important but these are crucial. **Grape seed oil** is gentle and a good binding agent as well if you decide to make your own skin-firming substance. And take a good

multivitamin daily which includes as many of the vitamins and minerals listed above as possible. These are good first steps at firming skin. Of course, if you have cellulite, add the cellulite-fighting substances like **caffeine** crème and **apple cider vinegar** as well. A sensible approach is to test and incorporate each new substance one by one so that if a reaction occurs, you will immediately know which new substance to avoid.

This dual approach of taking these critical substances as supplements and of using them as external applications directly on our skin has a great chance of building the collagen we need to support our connective tissue in doing its job—connecting our loose skin back to its underlying muscle tissue.

Treatments by Target

Collagen Support
- vitamin A/retinol
- amino acids: lysine plus L-arginine
- bioflavonoids
- vitamin C
- vitamin E
- ellagic acid
- glucosamine
- gotu kola
- kinetin
- manganese
- methylsulfonylmethane (MSM)
- seaweed extract/fucoxanthin
- silica

Connective Tissue Support
- vitamin A/beta-carotene
- amino acids: alanine, creatine, L-carnitine, and L-ornithine
- vitamin B-2
- copper peptides
- vitamin E
- hyaluronic acid
- punicalagin
- zinc

Lymphatic Support
- aescin
- vitamin B-6

Cellulite Reduction
- apple cider vinegar
- caffeine
- cocoa butter
- grape seed oil
- green tea extract
- seaweed extract/fucoxanthin

Skin Support
- alpha-hydroxy acids
- alpha lipoic acids
- antioxidants
- vitamin B-3
- beta-hydroxy acid/salicylic acid
- mustard oil
- lycopene
- fish oil (EPA)
- quercetin
- resveratrol
- seabuckthorn
- selenium

Muscle Support
- calcium

Recommended Daily Allowances

1 g = 1,000 mg (.001 g) = 1,000,000 mcg (.001 mg)

Supplement/ Crème	RDA (Females 18-65)	RDA (Males 18-65)	Suggested or Sample Daily Amount[1]	Potential Side Effects/Other Precautions[2]
Vitamin A/Beta-Carotene Supplement	700 mcg	900 mcg	RDA	1500+ mcg may increase cancer risk if you smoke, drink alcohol heavily or have been exposed to asbestos.
Vitamin A/Retinol Crème	n/a	n/a	30-60 mg per oz	May cause peeling, redness, skin warmth, irritation, sensitivity to sunlight, stinging, nausea, dry skin, muscle pain. Rarely, may cause severe allergic reaction.
Aescin Supplement/ Crème	n/a	n/a	400-650 mg	Do not use if you have edema (swelling).
Aloe Vera Gel	n/a	n/a	100%	No significant side effects.
Alpha Hydroxy Acids Crème	n/a	n/a	85%	May cause skin irritation, redness, dryness; may increase sensitivity to sunlight. Rarely, may cause severe allergic

---

[1] Use common sense. This book does not constitute medical advice. Do not add *any* supplement or nutrient in *any* amount to your diet, particularly if you are on any medication, prescription or otherwise, or if you have any health concerns whatsoever, until you speak to your physician. Do not take these or any supplements if pregnant or nursing unless your doctor tells you to!

[2] Typically, severe and/or allergic reactions are rare. Speak to your physician or dermatologist before putting any external substance on your skin. Test any new external substance in an inconspicuous spot on your body, such as in the fold of your elbow, before putting it on your face or slathering it on your body. Never put any substance on your face until you've tested it elsewhere on your body! Discontinue use immediately if you experience a reaction or adverse side effects.

				reactions.
Alpha Lipoic Acids Supplement	n/a	n/a	200 mg	May lower blood sugar.
Amino Acids				
• Alanine Supplement	n/a	n/a	200-600 mg	600+ g may damage liver or kidneys.
• Creatine Supplement	n/a	n/a	10 g	High doses may cause kidney damage.
• L-Carnitine Supplement	n/a	n/a	1-3 g	5+ g may cause stomach upset, impair thyroid, increase blood pressure, impair blood clotting, decrease appetite.
• Lysine + L-Arginine Supplement	n/a	n/a	1000 mg	High doses may cause gallstones.
• L-Ornithine Supplement	n/a	n/a	500 mg at bedtime	Do not exceed 10+ g.
Apple Cider Vinegar	n/a	n/a	100%	Rarely, may cause throat pain, allergic reactions, hives, difficulty breathing; may cause tissue irritation with extended use.
Vitamin B				
• B-2/Riboflavin Supplement	1.1 mg	1.3 mg	RDA	10+ mg may cause eye damage in bright sunlight.
• B-3/ Niacin Supplement	14 mg	16 mg	RDA	50+ mg may cause heat flushes, liver damage, stomach ulcers.
• B-6/Pyridoxine Supplement	1.3 mg	1.3 mg	RDA	100+ mg may cause nerve damage.
Beta-Hydroxy Acid/ Salicylic Acid Crème	n/a	n/a	30%	May cause skin irritation, redness and dryness.
Bioflavonoids Supplement	n/a	n/a	250 mg	May elevate estrogen levels; may cause allergic reactions

				(vomiting, nausea, rash).
Vitamin C/Ascorbic Acid Supplement	75 mg	90 mg	RDA	2000+ mg may cause diarrhea, gas, stomach upset
Vitamin C/L-Ascorbic Acid Serum	n/a	n/a	25% (begin with a milder solution to avoid irritation)	May cause skin irritation, redness, itching, dryness.
Caffeine Crème	n/a	n/a	5+% or 1/3rd cup fresh grounds if homemade	No significant side effects.
Calcium Supplement	1000 mg	1000 mg	RDA	High doses may cause constipation and stomach upset, kidney damage, irregular heart rhythm.
Cocoa Butter Crème	n/a	n/a	100%	May cause allergic reactions (swelling, hives, itching, skin rashes); may exacerbate adult acne.
Co-enzyme Q10/Ubiquinol Supplement	30-200 mg	30-200 mg	RDA	High doses may cause stomach upset; may lower blood sugar.
Copper Peptides Crème	n/a	n/a	.1+%	May cause redness, burning, rashes, skin inflammation. Do not take internally.
Vitamin E Supplement	15 mg/ 22.4 IU	15 mg/ 22.4 IU	RDA	High doses may thin blood. May interact with medications including antidepressants, antipsychotics, cancer drugs, etc.
Vitamin E Crème or Oil	n/a	n/a	10,000 IU	May cause inflammation, redness, itchiness, swelling.
Ellagic Acid Supplement	n/a	n/a	40-900 mg	May increase blood pressure.
Fish Oil (EPA not DHA) Supplement	180 mg	180 mg	RDA	May thin blood. May cause bloating, gas and diarrhea.

Glucosamine Supplement	1500 mg	1500 mg	RDA	May cause stomach upset, diarrhea. May raise blood pressure and cholesterol levels.
Gotu Kola Supplement	1000-4000 mg	1000-4000 mg	RDA	May affect the liver. May cause skin allergies, headache, stomach upset, drowsiness. Do not use if you have a history of cancerous or precancerous skin lesions.
Grape Seed Extract	n/a	n/a	50-100 mg	May cause headache, nausea, dizziness, dry skin, dry scalp. May thin blood.
Green Tea Extract	100-750 mg	100-750 mg	RDA	May cause irritability, insomnia, heart palpitations, dizziness.
Hyaluronic Acid/Glycos-aminoglycan Serum	n/a	n/a	100%	May cause slight skin reactions.
Kinetin Crème	n/a	n/a	.03-.1%	May cause allergic reactions (hives, rash, difficulty breathing, swelling).
Lycopene Supplement	10-30 mg	10-30 mg	RDA	May irritate stomach ulcers. May cause stomach upset.
Manganese Supplement	1.8 mg	2.3 mg	RDA	10+ mg may cause nervous system damage, loss of appetite, headaches, leg cramps, tremors, convulsions, irritability, violence, hallucinations.
Methylsulfonyl-methane (MSM) Supplement	n/a	n/a	2-6 g	May cause allergic reactions, nausea, diarrhea, headache, fatigue.
Quercetin Supplement	n/a	n/a	200-500 mg	1+ g may damage kidneys. May cause

				diarrhea, headache, stomach upset.
Resveratrol Supplement	n/a	n/a	100-500 mg	Do not take if you have or are at high risk for breast cancer.
Seabuckthorn Extract/Oil (cold-pressed)	n/a	n/a	500 mg or 300 ml	May interact with other medications. May cause temporary yellowing of skin.
Seaweed Extract/ Fucoxanthin	n/a	n/a	100-1000 mg	May thin blood. May increase iodine levels; avoid if taking thyroid medication. Excessive amounts may cause yellowing of skin.
Selenium Supplement	55 mcg	55 mcg	RDA	200+ mcg may increase the risk of developing diabetes. Do not take if you have an underactive thyroid or are at risk for skin cancer. High doses may cause fingernail loss, skin rash, fatigue, irritability, weight loss.
Silica (Horsetail) Supplement	900 mg	900 mg	RDA	Do not use if you have heart or kidney disorders, diabetes or gout. Do not drink alcohol heavily. Do not use with nicotine patches or nicotine gum.
Zinc Supplement	8 mg	11 mg	RDA	40+ mg may cause dizziness, headache, drowsiness, sweating, loss of muscle coordination, alcohol intolerance, hallucinations, anemia. May raise cholesterol.

Skin-Tightening Internal Supplements

- vitamin A/beta-carotene
- aescin
- alpha lipoic acids
- amino acids (alanine, creatine, L-carnitine, lysine and L-arginine, L-ornithine)
- vitamin B (B-2, B-3, B-6)
- bioflavonoids
- vitamin C/ascorbic acid
- calcium
- co-enzyme Q10
- vitamin E
- ellagic acid
- glucosamine
- gotu kola
- grape seed extract
- green tea extract
- lycopene
- manganese
- methylsulfonylmethane (MSM)
- fish oil (EPA not DHA)
- quercetin
- resveratrol
- seabuckthorn
- seaweed extract/fucoxanthin
- selenium
- silica/horsetail
- zinc

Skin-Tightening Crèmes, Lotions, Oils and External Treatments Ingredients

- vitamin A/retinol
- aescin
- aloe vera gel
- alpha-hydroxy acids or beta-hydroxy acid/salicylic acid
- vitamin C/L-ascorbic acid
- caffeine
- cocoa butter
- co-enzyme Q10
- copper peptides
- vitamin E
- grape seed oil/mustard oil
- green tea
- hyaluronic acid/glycosaminoglycan serum
- kinetin
- punicalagin
- seabuckthorn oil
- (any other substance listed on the Internal Supplements list)

Skin-Tightening Superfoods

Fruits & Berries
- apples (ellagic acid)
- apricots (bioflavonoids)
- black currants (antioxidants, bioflavonoids)
- blackberries (antioxidants, ellagic acid)
- blueberries (antioxidants, ellagic acid)
- cantaloupe (vitamin A)
- cherries (bioflavonoids, ellagic acid)
- concord grapes (antioxidants)
- cranberries (ellagic acid)
- currants (vitamin B-2)
- dried fruits (calcium)
- elderberries (bioflavonoids)
- fruit (silica)
- Goji berries (vitamin C)
- grapefruit (bioflavonoids)
- grapes (bioflavonoids, ellagic acid)
- guava (lycopene)
- hawthorn berry (bioflavonoids)
- kiwi (vitamin C)
- mangoes (vitamin A)
- oranges and citrus fruits (vitamin C, bioflavonoids, calcium)
- papaya (vitamins A & C, lycopene)
- peaches (vitamin A, ellagic acid)
- pink grapefruit (lycopene)
- plums (antioxidants)
- pomegranates (vitamins A & C, ellagic acid, punicalagin)
- prunes (bioflavonoids)

- purple figs (antioxidants)
- red raspberries (ellagic acid, punicalagin)
- strawberries (ellagic acid)
- watermelon (vitamin C, lycopene)

Vegetables

- argula (calcium)
- asparagus (vitamin E)
- avocados (vitamins B-2 & E, manganese)
- beets (antioxidants)
- bell peppers (vitamin C)
- broccoli (vitamins B-2 & C, calcium, co-enzyme Q10, omega 3 fatty acids)
- Brussels sprouts (vitamin C)
- carrots (vitamins A & B-3)
- collard greens (vitamin A)
- corn (vitamin B-3)
- dark green leafy vegetables (amino acids, vitamin B-2, calcium, manganese, omega 3 fatty acids)
- eggplant (antioxidants)
- horsetail (bioflavonoids)
- kale (vitamins A, C & E, calcium)
- leeks (MSM)
- mushrooms (selenium, zinc)
- onions (MSM)
- peppers (bioflavonoids)
- pumpkin (vitamin A)
- purple cabbage (antioxidants)
- red bell peppers (lycopene)
- red carrots (lycopene)
- shallots (MSM)
- spinach (vitamin A & C, omega 3 fatty acids)

- sun dried tomatoes (copper)
- tomatoes (copper, lycopene)

Eggs & Dairy

- cheese (amino acids, calcium, vitamins B-2 & B-3, zinc)
- cow's milk (calcium, MSM)
- dairy products (vitamins A, B-2, B-3 & B-6, amino acids, calcium)
- egg whites (zinc)
- eggs (vitamins A, B-2, B-6 & E, amino acids, manganese, protein, selenium)
- soy milk (calcium)

Meat

- beef (vitamin B-3)
- beef liver (co-enzyme Q10)
- chicken (amino acids, vitamin B-6, co-enzyme Q10, protein)
- ground beef (amino acids)
- kidneys (vitamin B-6)
- lamb (amino acids, zinc)
- liver (vitamin B-6, copper, manganese)
- meats (amino acids)
- organ meats (vitamin B-2)
- pork (amino acids, vitamins B-3 & B-6, co-enzyme Q10)
- turkey (selenium)

Seafood

- calamari (copper)
- catfish (amino acids)
- cod (amino acids, protein)

- crab (copper, protein)
- fish (amino acids, vitamins B-2, B-3 & B-6, omega 3 fatty acids)
- lobster (copper, protein)
- mackerel (co-enzyme Q10)
- oysters (copper, selenium, zinc)
- salmon (calcium, omega 3 fatty acids)
- sardines (amino acids, zinc)
- shellfish (copper)
- shrimp (selenium)
- tahini (copper)
- yellowtail tuna (co-enzyme Q10)

Soy, Beans & Lentils

- beans (amino acids, calcium, copper, zinc)
- chickpeas (amino acids)
- kidney beans (amino acids)
- lentils (amino acids, zinc)
- navy beans (amino acids)
- soy (amino acids, resveratrol)
- soy milk (calcium)
- soybeans (co-enzyme Q10, copper)
- tofu (calcium, zinc)

Cereals, Grains & Starches

- brewer's yeast (vitamin B-6)
- brown rice (manganese)
- buckwheat (bioflavonoids)
- cereal grains (amino acids)
- oatmeal (calcium)
- pasta (selenium)
- potatoes (vitamin B-3)

- sweet potatoes (vitamin A)
- wheat germ (vitamin B-6)
- whole grains (manganese, silica, zinc)
- whole wheat (vitamin B-3)

Oils & Vinegars

- apple cider vinegar
- canola oil (co-enzyme Q10)
- fish oil (omega 3 fatty acids)
- olive oil (resveratrol)
- palm oil (vitamin A)
- vegetable oils (vitamin E)

Nuts & Seeds

- almonds (calcium, copper, vitamin E, manganese)
- Brazil nuts (selenium)
- dried nuts (calcium)
- chia seeds (calcium)
- flax seeds or flax seed oil (calcium, omega 3 fatty acids)
- hazelnuts (copper)
- hemp (omega 3 fatty acids)
- nuts (amino acids, vitamin B-2, co-enzyme Q10, copper)
- pecans (ellagic acid)
- pistachios (copper)
- pumpkin seeds (copper, zinc)
- roasted squash seeds (copper)
- sesame seeds (calcium, copper)
- sunflower and other seeds (calcium, copper, vitamin E, selenium)
- walnuts (ellagic acid, manganese, omega 3 fatty acids)
- quinoa (amino acids, calcium)

Herbs & Spices
- chervil (bioflavonoids)
- chives (MSM)
- cinnamon (resveratrol)
- dried herbs (calcium, copper)
- garlic (MSM)
- oregano (resveratrol)
- parsley (co-enzyme Q10)
- rosehips (bioflavonoids, lycopene)
- spices (manganese)

Coffee & Tea
- coffee (manganese, resveratrol)
- green tea (antioxidants)
- tea (manganese, quercetin, resveratrol)

Etc.
- blackstrap molasses (calcium)
- seaweed/wakame/hijiki (vitamins A, C & E, amino acids, antioxidants, calcium, fucoxanthin, protein)
- unsweetened cocoa powder (copper)
- yeast (vitamin B-2)

4

Skin-Tightening Exercises

This book focuses on ways to get our loose skin to adhere to the underlying muscle via the connective tissue. We have thoroughly examined our skin and our connective tissue. Let's now turn to the foundation piece–the underlying muscle. Get ready to lift weights, baby!

When we diet and as we age, our muscle mass decreases unless we take specific measures to prevent it. Furthermore, you may not even have that much muscle mass to begin with if you haven't already taken steps to increase it through a lifetime of targeted physical activity. Personally, I never lifted weights on any schedule or with any intensity until about four years ago. I didn't want to bulk up. But I started lifting weights in my late 30s and it has made a major positive difference both in my health and my body.

Aerobic exercise–cardio–that seeks to burn fat and increase health through repetitive activities generally performed at light, moderate or intensive pace, or as high-intensity intervals, is great for your health and fitness. It helps burn fat and may decrease cellulite, which is important, but it doesn't specifically build the quantity of muscle mass we need to give our loose skin a good foundation to adhere to.

To build muscle, you must lift weights. More specifically, you must lift heavy weights.

Build a Firm Foundation With Heavy Lifting

Some people, women in particular, fear becoming massive, hulking "he-women" if they work out with heavy weights and/or use free weights—dumbbells or barbells—instead of machines. That's virtually impossible unless that is your specific intent and you undertake many accompanying steps, like special supplements and even steroids to accomplish this. Many women who do lift weights restrict themselves to very light weights—1-, 2-, 5- or 10-pound weights—because they are afraid of bulking up, afraid of injury or they simply think they can't lift anything heavier.

Nothing could be further from the truth.

Obviously, if you're not accustomed to lifting heavy weights, or to lifting weights at all, you probably aren't going to walk into a gym and pop off five sets of 50 pound bicep curls. It's something that needs to be worked up to gradually and safely. (And I'm not suggesting that most women specifically want or need to perform 50 pound bicep curls—but hey, if you can, great!)

The best resource I've found on this topic is a set of books, *The New Rules of Lifting* (which is the men's version), and *The New Rules of Lifting for Women*.

I've included a few suggested exercises I use below, but to really understand the physiology behind the heavy-lifting method, and for specific workouts that target the muscles we want to build in our upper arms, thighs, buttocks, back and abdomen—where the loose skin generally hangs out—I strongly encourage you to invest in *The New Rules* written for your gender. It's a wonderful book—clear, concise and very well written—and it breaks down everything you need to know to build the muscles your firming skin needs to adhere to. You should be able to find it at your local bookstore, on Amazon.com, or wherever you typically buy books.

In the interim, the approach I've found that works best for me is to perform as many reps (repetitions, or the number of times you can repeat a move)—which ends up being a very small number—as I can, using the highest weight I can.

As an example, for bicep curls specifically, this tends to be three sets of three reps using 35-pound dumbbells. This means, I do three bicep curls at 35 pounds, rest for a minute, repeat, rest for a minute, repeat. That's the maximum weight I can lift for this particular exercise at this time, and I can only lift it nine total times (sometimes less) before I give out. It's a fair amount of weight for a woman to lift.

I couldn't use the 35-pound weights when I seriously started lifting weights four years ago. It was a struggle even to lift one off the rack using both hands. It took a long time to work up to actually using them. But I was serious about it, and, over time, I was able to lift heavier weights.

The New Rules recommends three total-body workouts (all major muscle groups) per week, with recovery time between each exercise, and also with a full day of recovery between each workout. It also has suggestions for diet, which I don't follow because it's too carb-intensive for me, but it's a sound nutrition plan, if you're looking for one. It has other recommendations as well, like keeping a training log to track your progress.

These books truly are the best resource you can use to lay the muscle foundation you need to firm your skin. In general, some exercises you can do to help build muscle include:

- chest presses
- crunches on a Swiss ball
- deadlifts
- lateral pulldowns
- lunges
- pectoral flies
- planks
- push-ups
- shoulder presses
- squats

If you aren't ready to invest in *The New Rules* or a similar program, you can search the Internet for good instructions on how to do the exercises listed above and others, safely, correctly and effectively.

You may also want to incorporate some work with machines in addition to the free weights, but do not avoid free weights altogether in favor of only using machines, or you will not get the results you want to see.

And the key is–lift heavy weights, not light weights. Don't let a well-meaning friend or personal trainer talk you out of heavy weights, either. You aren't going to bulk up–that's a myth. And, another great thing about lifting heavy weights with a low number of repetitions is, it takes a lot less time out of your day than hours of light weight lifting, or hours of cardio, do. You can do more in less time and get much more gratifying results.

Further, it's helpful, but not necessary, to join a gym or to hire a personal trainer in order to see the kind of results we want to achieve in order to build the muscle layer underlying the skin we want to firm.

You can purchase a decent set of free weights and, if you like, a bench and a full-length mirror, at your local discount store (Target, Wal-Mart, etc.) or you often can find someone selling a set they no longer use online (try your local Craigslist) or in your local newspaper classifieds. All you want is the results–the setting in which you attain them really doesn't matter. Just make sure you're safe, comfortable and motivated. Don't let your weight bench become extra storage for clothes!

Above all, be safe and use common sense. Don't lift more than you can safely handle, otherwise you may injure yourself. Be very careful when handling heavy weights and have a safe place to store them where you, your kids and your pets can't accidentally get hurt. *Always* check with your physician before beginning *any* exercise program, particularly one that incorporates strenuous activity like heavy weight lifting. And know what you're doing before you begin, either by reading the books I recommend above or by consulting a personal trainer who subscribes to the heavy-lifting philosophy. Ask first before you hire them since many don't agree with this philosophy, instead supporting the more-traditional light weight lifting philosophy. There's nothing wrong with that philosophy; it's just not going to garner the results we want to achieve when our specific goal is to tighten loose skin.

Since we're doing all we can to strengthen our skin through our lymph system and to strengthen the connective tissue between our skin and our muscle, it only makes sense that we do all we can to strengthen the muscle beneath the skin as well. This three-pronged approach is our best bet for firming our loose skin and being able to trade that baggy t-shirt and shorts for a string bikini.

In addition to lifting heavy weights to build a good foundation of muscle underneath our skin, other exercises can be useful in strengthening our lymph systems and in improving the overall tone and appearance of our skin.

Rebounding

In 1980, scientists at the NASA Ames Research Center in California published a research paper in the *Journal of Applied Physiology* entitled "Body Acceleration Distribution and Oxygen Uptake in Humans During Running and Jumping." NASA had been working to find ways to keep astronauts from losing bone density, muscle mass and strength while in space, where they were losing strength and tone while outside the pull of gravity.

NASA tested many forms of exercise on the astronauts and found that one exercise was over two-thirds more efficient than walking on a treadmill or any other form of exercise: rebounding, or jumping on a mini trampoline.

Those studied reported that, not only did their health and energy improve, their skin glowed *and their saggy skin tightened up.* Why?

Rebounding on a mini trampoline supports, improves and benefits many systems in our bodies. Rebounding uses gravity through acceleration and deceleration.

When jumping on a trampoline, we experience a change in G force. G force is one unit of the force of gravity on the surface of the earth; it measures the force we experience during acceleration. We drop to a G force of nearly zero at the top of a trampoline jump and we reach a G force of approximately 1.5 when we bottom out on the trampoline. Furthermore, the G force is spread evenly throughout the body so jumping on a mini trampoline is a no-impact aerobic exercise.

Rebounding is great for our lymph systems. As we learned in Section 1, our circulatory system has blood vessels to circulate blood throughout our body with a built-in pump—our hearts. Our lymph systems, which circulate lymphatic fluid through the body, have no such pump. They rely on bodily movement to circulate lymph fluid.

Rebounding is a very good way to stimulate the circulation of our lymph systems. Lack of G force at the top of a jump opens our lymph valves, heavier G force at the bottom of a jump closes them, and the movement in between pushes the lymph fluid through the lymph system itself. A badly functioning lymph system shows in the condition of our skin and a well-functioning lymph system helps our skin as much as anything can.

Rebounding stresses cells, including skin cells. This sounds bad but it's not. Cells and cell walls that are stressed through rebounding grow firmer and stronger. The more they continue to be stressed, the stronger and firmer they become. The effects of jumping on a mini trampoline are cumulative—the longer we jump, over time, the better our results.

The other really great advantage to jumping on a mini trampoline is—it's fun! It doesn't seem like exercise, it seems like you're sneaking off to jump on your bed while Mom isn't looking. It's an almost-no-impact exercise that virtually anyone can do.

Mini trampoline prices start at about $25 at local discount stores or you can find better-quality ones online or at your local sporting goods store. To save time, you can also check out a variety of rebounders on this book's Amazon.com store: http://astore.amazon.com/firlooski-20.

I bought a perfectly serviceable mini trampoline at my local sporting goods store for about $50, weight tested up to 200 pounds. I wanted to test this wacky-sounding skin-firming theory out before investing a lot in a high-quality rebounder, and my excitement with the results I'm already seeing after only a few weeks was part of what led me to write this book.

My inexpensive mini trampoline won't last forever and I've already decided that my next one will be a better-quality upgrade. Rebounding definitely helps skin and I strongly encourage you to invest in one.

Be sure that any rebounder you buy has a quality guarantee and is weight-tested to hold you. Mini trampolines can be found that hold up to 400 pounds or more. Also, rebounders can be ordered online that come with a stability bar, so even if you're less steady on your feet you can still jump safely and securely.

Don't overtax yourself when you're first starting out. Jump for a couple of minutes then take a break. Eventually you should be able to work your way up to 20 minutes or more. It's an easy exercise but it does take a lot of effort–don't overdo it, or you'll be sore the next day.

Typically, most experts advise jumping at least 20 minutes a day. This can be done easily if you break it up into two 10-minute sessions, one in the morning, one at night. You can even get mini trampolines that fold for storage and travel. There also are videos on YouTube and available for sale online which show you different exercises and programs you can follow while jumping for various types of results, and so you don't get bored with it.

Two warnings: if you are prone to detached retinas, don't jump on a mini trampoline until you clear it with your eye doctor. And, if you have weak ankles or other foot or ankle problems, again, talk to your doctor or podiatrist before jumping on a rebounder. As with any exercise, it's a good idea to run it past your doctor and get a general checkup before starting any exercise program—particularly if you are out of shape.

Even if you act on no other recommendation or idea from this book, *please* buy a mini trampoline and jump on it. I've been jumping for several months now and I'm starting to see some results. There are testimonials galore on the Internet that this works. It's good for your skin and for the rest of you, too.

Foam Roller Exercises

One technique that seems to be gaining in popularity claims to increase circulation, break up fat and reduce cellulite by using a foam roller to deeply massage the areas of our bodies where cellulite accumulates—hips, legs, thighs, buttocks, abdomen, etc.

Foam rollers have been used for rehabilitation from injuries for years. Rolling out your legs, back, buttocks and other large muscle groups increases blood circulation and oxygen flow to those areas. Fitness experts recommend rolling out hips, thighs and buttocks 15-20 minutes at a time, three times a week.

To perform this exercise, lie sideways on the foam roller and roll back and forth over it, concentrating on your inner and outer thighs, hips and buttocks. A quick Internet search will bring up photos and examples of this interesting approach to cellulite reduction.

Working Out From the Neck Up

The skin on our faces and necks can sag due to tanning, smoking, weight loss or aging. Obviously we can't lift heavy weights to firm this skin but there are some targeted exercises we can do that many people claim helps firm face and neck skin, at least to some extent.

For many of us, our chins, necks and faces start to wrinkle and sag over the age of 40. A reduction in collagen frequently is the culprit—so, following the suggestions in the previous section to increase collagen production from the inside through supplements and superfoods, and from the outside with targeted crèmes and lotions, should help a lot in improving our skin's collagen production. Exercising these areas may help as well.

Facial and neck exercises work to improve blood flow and to oxygenate, strengthen and tone the muscles and firm the skin. Exercises targeted to these areas have worked for some in firming up sagging chins and necks.

A few of the more popular ones, which should be done several times each day for the best effect, include the following. Note that you probably won't want to do these exercises in front of friends and family unless they, and you, have a really good sense of humor. They look silly! But some report that they do make a difference—so have fun with them.

These exercises are most comfortably done in a seated position, in a sturdy chair with back support. For each of the exercises below, start out with a few reps and work your way up to more sets. Believe it or not, your face, chin and neck will get tired after just a few to start. Don't overdo it or you may experience soreness the next day.

These exercises are best performed at least once a day, preferably twice. Hold each position below for a count of five then relax for another count of five before performing the next one.

Surprise! and **Cat's Meow**: Open mouth and eyes as widely as you can simultaneously (and gently). Hold for a few seconds then relax and repeat. Open mouth again widely and stick out tongue. These are good stretches to get the blood flowing in the neck and face.

Forehead Push/Pull: Place the heels of your hands flat against your forehead. Push your forehead firmly against your hands and keep your hands in place, so your forehead doesn't have anywhere to go. You will feel your neck muscles flex. Hold for a few seconds then relax and repeat. Clasp your hands behind your head, and push back, again not letting your head move. Hold for a few seconds then relax and repeat. These exercises strengthen your neck muscles, front and back.

Anti-Eyeliner: Squint and release eyes. Hold for a few seconds then relax and repeat. This strengthens muscles under the eyes to reduce puffiness and lines. Remember, however, that you always want to wear sunglasses when you're outside to avoid squinting all day long. Too much squinting causes crow's feet.

Eyebrow Raise: Place a finger above each eyebrow. Raise your eyebrows while pressing down with your fingers. Hold for a few seconds then repeat. Push down with your fingers while raising your eyebrows. Hold for a few seconds then repeat. These exercises decrease horizontal lines on your forehead and vertical frown lines over the bridge of your nose.

Kiss the Sky: Tilt you head backwards until you are looking straight upwards. Pull your lips back into a big grin, showing teeth, hold for a few seconds, then purse your lips as though you are trying to kiss the sky. Hold for a few seconds then relax and repeat.

Kiss Your Nose: Purse your lips tightly then raise them towards your nose. Hold for a few seconds then relax and repeat. This helps increase the fullness of lips.

Hollow/Full Cheeks: Suck your cheeks in. Hold for a few seconds then relax. Fill your cheeks full of air to stretch them out. Hold for a few seconds then relax and repeat. This exercise helps strengthen the cheek and facial muscles.

Tongue Press: Tilt your head back so you're looking straight up. Press your tongue against the roof of your mouth. Lower your head until you're looking straight forward. Hold for a few seconds then relax and repeat. This helps smooth out the skin on your jawline.

Chin Push: Tilt your head back so you're looking straight up. Stick your chin out as far as you can. Hold for a few seconds then relax and repeat. This helps smooth out the skin on your neck.

Chin Raise: Raise your bottom lip over your upper lip as though you have an underbite then tilt your head back so you're looking straight up. Wait a beat, then stick your tongue out downwardly as though you're trying to lick your chin. Hold for a few seconds then relax and repeat. You can really feel the pull in the skin over your throat on this one and it targets the area where excess fat tends to accrue.

By the way, sitting in your car in traffic is a great place to do these exercises. If the driver of the next car gives you a funny look, just smile and wave.

5

Other Non-Surgical Treatments

Recent advances in non-surgical skin techniques have come a long way. Surgical intervention now is not the only way to tighten skin when less-invasive techniques don't do the job.

The following section presents a brief sample of other non-surgical skin-tightening techniques. When considering any technique, be sure to seek out trained, licensed professionals, get second opinions (or more), know the risks, possible complications and possible side effects, and be sure you get a realistic assessment of how much any particular procedure may help, how many sessions you may need, how long positive effects may last (many are not permanent), and perform a cost/benefit analysis of how much you're willing to spend versus possibility of success versus how long effects are expected to last.

What many of these procedures target is the collagen layer, seeking to build it up by various means. This is *precisely* what we are trying to do with the other techniques in this book, particularly with skin-firming supplements and external treatments, at far less cost and virtually no danger or discomfort. Consider supplements first, these treatments second.

Typically, non-surgical techniques aren't going to be as effective or long-lasting as surgical procedures. They carry their own risks as well, including the risk of pain, permanent scarring, or of noticeably lightening your wallet without noticeably tightening your skin. But there are still some old-fashioned, tried-and-true techniques that may be just as effective and far less costly. My favorite among these is dry skin brushing.

Dry Skin Brushing

Dry brushing skin is fast, easy and it feels great. The only item needed is a long-handled soft-bristled brush, typically available inexpensively at any store that sells beauty or bath supplies, discount store or online at places such as Amazon.com.

Some claim the lymph-stimulating results on cellulite of daily dry brushing of skin is equivalent to 30 minutes a day of aerobic exercise. Dry skin brushing claims to stimulate the lymph system by helping lymphatic fluid move throughout the body and proponents claim dry skin brushing works to eliminate cellulite and tighten skin healthfully and naturally.

A number of methods and recommendations exist for "proper" dry brushing, but the three key principles to remember are, always brush towards your heart, don't brush too hard, and clean your brush often (you can take it in the shower with you, wash it with shampoo and let it air-dry naturally).

Begin brushing either at your hands or feet. Brush briskly yet gently (if it's uncomfortable, you're doing it too hard–this should feel wonderful and relaxing). Starting with your fingertips or toes, use brisk long brushstrokes and brush inwards towards your heart.

From the fingertips, brush the backs of your hands, then the palms, forearms up to your elbows, then elbows to shoulders. From the feet, brush the tops and soles of your feet up to your ankles, ankles upward to knees, knees to thighs, upwards to the buttocks, up the bottom half of your back, down the back from the shoulders to the waist, downwards from the shoulders to the chest, up the abdomen to the heart, and then very gently downwards on your face, throat and neck. Always brush towards your heart since that's the direction lymph fluid flows.

Once you get into the habit of this it only takes about two minutes a day and it's very invigorating. The best time to dry brush is right before you take a shower.

Non-Surgical Cosmetic Procedures

Ablative Fractionated Carbon Dioxide (CO₂) Laser: Also called a "laser eyelift," typically the ablative fractioned CO_2 laser is used to treat sun-damaged skin and to tighten loose skin around the eyes. Side effects typically are minimal and may include lost time from work, pain, swelling, burns, scarring or other complications. Most risks occur due to infection. Repeatedly lasing the same area is not advised as it increases the chances of scarring. People with dark-pigmented skin are advised to use cautiously. Expect to spend several thousand dollars on this procedure.

Broad-Spectrum Light Sources: The use of a broad-spectrum light source is a non-surgical, non-invasive skin-tightening treatment which uses a broad band of infrared light (typically 850-1800 nanometers) to heat the middle layer of skin to encourage new collagen to grow. Some patients' skin tightens visibly after only one treatment, others need more and they will notice a more-gradual tightening of the skin. The skin-tightening effect ordinarily is not permanent but generally does last at least 12 months. Costs may start at about $300 or more per session; multiple sessions often are needed.

Collagen Injections: Typically targeting the face, collagen can be injected directly under the skin to provide a smoother, less-wrinkled appearance. Effects ordinarily last a few months then must be repeated. Prices typically start at well under $1000.

Focused Ultrasound (Ulthera): Ulthera, like laser treatments, uses ultrasound to target the middle layer of skin to encourage collagen to grow. Some patients may experience a good bit of discomfort during the procedure. Results may take several months to become apparent and tend to last 2-3 years, on average.

Mesotherapy: This treatment targets cellulite with injections of small quantities of vitamins, plant extracts and other substances under the skin. Common side effects include stinging at the site, soreness and bruising. Expect to pay a couple thousand dollars for this treatment which seems to have mixed reviews.

Unipolar and Monopolar Radiofrequency: Unipolar radiofrequency is used to treat cellulite and monopolar radiofrequency, or Thermage, is used to tighten skin on the face, neck and body. Unipolar radiofrequency claims to be a very effective cellulite treatment and scientific studies seem to back this up. Thermage is growing in popularity due to recent improvements in results and reduction in side effects, including less pain and discomfort. This procedure also heats deeper layers of skin to encourage collagen production while cooling the outer layers. The majority of Thermage patients seem satisfied with the results and results may last 1-3 years, after which treatment must be repeated. Expect to pay several thousand dollars for either procedure.

The list above is just a sample of available cosmetic procedures and most are used primarily for loose skin on the face and secondarily the body. As with anything, check with your doctor and/or your dermatologist before deciding on any laser or other procedure to use. Know the risks and the probable effects, balance these against the costs, and make an informed decision.

Detoxification

Claims are out there purporting detoxes to be effective ways to reduce cellulite and/or flush the lymph system. There seems to be no hard scientific evidence that this works, but if detoxing is something you're drawn to, it probably won't hurt if practiced safely and intelligently and it may help, at least to some extent.

Liver Flushes

One particular detox some recommend is a liver flush/coffee enema. Typically a coffee enema incorporates a couple tablespoons of fresh coffee grounds in a quart of filtered water boiled on a stove in a non-aluminum pot.

Bring mixture to a boil, boil over low heat for five minutes, allow to cool to body temperature (add ice cubes if necessary), then strain through a fine strainer or cheesecloth to ensure all coffee grounds are removed.

Follow a typical enema process using the mixture at body temperature and retain the enema for 10-15 minutes if possible before expelling. You can easily search YouTube for video instructions on how to perform this or similar detox procedures.

Do not practice this enema more than once a week and do not perform more than three total coffee enemas without giving your body a long rest period. Definitely check with your doctor before you undertake this or any detox procedure.

Castor Oil Packs

Another liver and lymph system detox some claim works is a castor oil pack. Castor oil packs are purported to detox the liver, having a positive effect both on the health of the lymph system and on the appearance of cellulite throughout the body.

Castor oil packs are easy to make and to use, although they can be a bit messy. To make one, you will need:

- a bottle of castor oil (available in the stomach remedy aisle of your local pharmacy or online);
- flannel cloth (you can cut up an old flannel sheet);
- plastic wrap or unused trash bags;
- an old bath towel or two;

- a heating pad; and,
- some dampened paper towels.

For this detox, you will lie down, place the castor oil pack high on your abdomen, cover it with a heating pad, then relax for 30-to-90 minutes.

Cut the flannel into one-foot by one-foot squares. Saturate three squares with castor oil then heat them in a microwave-safe dish in your microwave until they are very warm, but not hot, to the touch. Wring them out well so that they are saturated but not dripping before using.

Spread an old bath towel down on your bed or sofa to lie on—you definitely don't want to get castor oil on your sheets or furniture. When you have all your supplies close by, remove your shirt, lay down on the bath towel, place the three stacked flannel cloths on your upper abdomen (the center of the pack should be over your liver, above and to the right of your belly button), cover the flannel pack with a sheet of plastic (plastic wrap or an unusued trash bag works great for this), place your heating pad turned on medium-high to high over the plastic sheeting, then cover your midsection with another bath towel, tucking it in on both sides to retain heat. The plastic sheeting will keep the castor oil from coming into contact with your heating pad and also helps retain heat.

Use damp paper towels to wipe any castor oil residue off your hands as needed while you lie back and relax during the treatment. You can do a castor oil pack while watching T.V. or reading a book. You may want to shower right afterwards—castor oil is very oily and may stain your clothing.

Typically, castor oil packs are used every other day for a week, or three days in a row followed by a four-day break. Save your castor oil-soaked flannel to reuse and store the remaining castor oil and used flannels in a Ziploc baggie in your refrigerator.

Some who have used castor oil packs report that, over time, the flannel will turn dark and crusty with the toxins that are drawn out of the liver and skin into it. Others have tried castor oil packs directly on cellulite-bearing areas, but few reports exist that this has any effect on cellulite. It's more likely to work as a liver detox than as a direct cellulite treatment, although it won't hurt to use a castor oil pack anywhere on the body. Note that, while castor oil used to be prescribed as an effective treatment for a variety of stomach ailments including constipation, now doctors advise that we ***not*** take castor oil internally. For external use only!

Compression Garments

Compression garments are used after abdominoplasty or other surgical skin-tightening procedures to help the remaining skin rebond to the underlying muscle tissue. But are they effective if you haven't had abdominal surgery?

If you have little or no fat remaining on your abdomen, thighs, upper arms or other body areas that have loose skin, theoretically, over time, a compression garment may help skin adhere to the underlying muscle. People who've had plastic surgery often are instructed to wear tight, surgical-grade compression garments on their arms, legs, thighs, abdomen or elsewhere depending on the area their surgery targeted. Various compression garments can be found on the Internet with a quick Google search, or less compressive garments, like Spanx, are available through many stores you may visit on a regular basis and through Amazon.com.

Anecdotally, I had a coworker at a previous job try this with mixed results. She had lost a good deal of weight and she decided to buy a firm corset-type girdle to see if it would help tighten the skin on her stomach. She wore it for several months and she thought it helped a little, but her husband thought it had made a big difference.

In theory, this could help if your body fat composition is very low but it may not be worth the discomfort. I remember how miserable my mother and grandmother were in the early

1970s when they wouldn't leave the house without a foundation garment. Girdles are not comfortable in anyone's book!

Wearing a compression garment may not be worth the discomfort since it's not a proven treatment for non-surgically treated loose skin–it might help, it might not. If you decide to go this route, I would suggest buying at least two quality garments that fit well, that compress firmly, and being cautious about the placement of your skin when you put one on. I recommend buying more than one so you'll have a clean one to wear while you launder the other.

I also wouldn't rely on this alone, but you might consider using it in addition to other methods suggested in this book, particularly the nutrition therapy through supplements, external treatments and superfoods as well as the heavy weight lifting, the rebounding, dry skin brushing and other proven treatments. And as always, you should consult your health care provider for advice first.

6

Real-Life Skin-Tightening Stories

I met Miranda, Melissa, Catherine and Prim through a weight loss discussion board on the Internet. The board has a section dedicated to discussing loose skin after weight loss and these women were gracious enough to share their personal weight loss and skin stories with me.

Miranda

Miranda is 21 years old and she has been losing weight for the past two years. She started out at over 250 pounds on a 5'6 frame and she has lost 85 pounds by counting calories and eating whole, unprocessed foods like the superfoods mentioned in section three. She has 15 pounds to go until she reaches her goal weight of 150 pounds. Miranda reports that she has no loose skin.

Miranda incorporates High-Intensity Interval Training (HIIT) with weight training, lifting heavy weights five-to-six times per week. Miranda's weight, fortunately, hasn't yo-yoed from high to low. Instead she gained slowly and steadily throughout the years until she decided it was time to lose the extra weight. She has never smoked or tanned on a regular basis and she has never had kids.

Despite losing 85 pounds, Miranda is fortunate that her skin has bounced back. Her young age and healthy lifestyle certainly help, but she credits the heavy weight lifting and plenty of exercise with her lack of loose skin. She advises others not to let the fear of loose skin discourage them from losing weight: "The benefits of weight loss far outweigh the chance that you might have some loose skin afterwards."

Melissa

Melissa is 42 years old, 5'6½ and currently weighs 172 pounds, having lost over 110 pounds in increments. Her greatest overall loss was in 2011 from a high weight of over 275 pounds. Her weight has yo-yoed over the years, losing 50, gaining 90, losing 40, gaining 30, then she got serious about it and she is maintaining her weight loss within 15 pounds of goal while working on getting to her final goal weight of 160. Melissa has loose skin.

Melissa avoids grains and tends to eat a balance of fats, protein and carbohydrates. She limits meat. Her ordinary diet comprises nuts and nut butter, a variety of vegetables, and apples. She exercises at least four days a week, doing step aerobics and Bodypump–a form of strength training to music that uses low weights with high numbers of repetitions. Her weight lifting philosophy is "Weight training just makes you look better and more fit." She has never smoked or tanned on a regular basis. She has had children–two of them–and she says her stomach is "one big stretch mark."

Melissa has loose skin on her upper arms, inner thighs, and particularly on her lower abdomen. She attributes most of this to the stretch marks from having kids and she thinks that having stretch marks is making it harder for her skin to bounce back.

She is convinced that nothing will help other than time, but she has made her peace with her loose skin and she calls it a "battle scar" from her war on weight. Her attitude to the loose skin is, "If it's the only reminder I have, besides photos, of my heavier self, then so be it."

Catherine

Catherine is 30 years old, 5'2, and she has lost a total of 62 pounds. She weighs 125, two pounds less than her original goal of 127 pounds. It took her seven months to lose the weight and she's spent the last six months working on toning. Her weight has never yo-yoed.

Her weight loss plan incorporates calorie counting and Volumetrics, which relies on foods with high water content like fruits and vegetables, soups, broths and stews, low-fat substitutes like skim milk and egg whites, lean protein, healthy fats, and drinking lots of water. She primarily eats whole foods and she mostly avoids processed foods. She doesn't smoke but she has tanned regularly since she was a teenager. Catherine has almost no loose skin but she does have stretch marks.

Catherine calls herself the "Zumba queen" and she also runs, rides her bike, takes an occasional kickboxing or yoga class and she has taken body sculpting classes that use light hand weights, typically in the five-to-15 pound range. She also strength trains using weight machines, using "enough weight to feel challenged but not overdo it."

She reports that she has very little loose skin but lots of stretch marks, which she attributes to having had two children. Catherine says, "The first pregnancy was what elevated my weight so much, and almost every stretch mark is from that initial pregnancy. My legs just lost all their elasticity."

She was very concerned about the possibility of loose skin when she began losing weight and it was that fear that kept her from losing weight for years. Her strategy for dealing with her skin has been to use a tinted daily moisturizer as a safe way to help camouflage her stretchmarks. Catherine says, "As I lost the weight, my legs did shrink. Not all the way, of course, but they tightened up very nicely. It was a very pleasant surprise."

Prim

Prim is 5'3 and she lost over 130 pounds in 2009. She is 42 years old, the same age as Melissa. Prim has maintained her new low weight for the last three years. From a high weight of 278 pounds, she currently weighs 145 and she would like to lose another 15. Prim was a regular yo-yo dieter, losing 20 pounds or more a handful of times and 50 pounds or more twice previously. Prim has some loose skin but she has incorporated many of the strategies put forth in this book to deal with them and she is hopeful that skin-tightening surgery will be unnecessary when she reaches goal weight.

To lose weight and maintain successfully this time, Prim has counted calories, beginning at 2000 per day and gradually lowering to her current 1500 per day. She limits processed food, grains, dairy and high-sugar fruits like bananas and grapes. She incorporates whole fats like olive oil, coconut oil and butter into her diet and she finds that this keeps her more satisfied and less prone to overeating than eating lower-fat foods did.

Her typical diet includes eggs and egg whites, beef, poultry and salmon, vegetables, citrus fruits and berries, almond milk, steel cut oatmeal, a variety of nuts and seeds, Greek yogurt and aged cheeses. She deals with her rare off-plan indulgences like pizza and fries with an intermittent fast, fasting for about a day then returning to her ordinary diet. She has never smoked or tanned on a regular basis and she has never had kids.

Prim exercises three-to-four days a week for 60-90 minutes. Like Miranda, she incorporates HIIT by attending a "boot camp" for 45 minutes, three days a week. She rides her bike periodically and she lifts heavy weights, to which she attributes much of her weight loss success. She also uses her downtime effectively, sometimes working out with resistance bands while watching T.V., but she doesn't do sit-ups: "I would do as many as 200 sit-ups a day and my stomach just bulged out more." Instead of sit-ups she performs planks and other core exercises as well as deep breathing to flatten her stomach, and she is pleased with the results.

Prim has loose skin on her upper arms, over her ribs and on her lower abdomen. She is very serious about getting rid of it.

Her strategy for dealing with loose skin, particularly with the loose skin on her upper arms, is to continue losing weight, with a goal of getting below 20% body fat. She also incorporates a variety of collagen-building and cellulite-fighting supplements and other activities into her extensive, daily weight loss and skin-firming regimen, including:

- a multivitamin
- fish oil
- magnesium
- biotin
- chromium
- St. John's wort
- green tea extract
- probiotics
- prebiotics
- branched chain amino acids
- two teaspoons of apple cider vinegar in eight ounces of water every morning
- a moisturizer
- dry skin brushing for 10 minutes prior to showering
- drinking water
- 20 minutes of weight training (almost) daily, concentrating on her arms

Prim isn't sure if she'll decide to have skin-tightening surgery after she reaches goal weight, but she hasn't ruled it out.

Heavy weight lifting seems to have helped Prim and Miranda. Concentrating on whole, natural, unprocessed foods seems to have helped all four women lose weight, and it likely has contributed to the health of their skin as well. All four have excellent attitudes towards loose skin and each has done an impressive job at losing weight and at maintaining their losses. Time alone will tell if Melissa's, Catherine's and Prim's loose skin tightens up as well as the youthful Miranda's did.

Prim's successes to date are remarkable. She is over 40 and she has lost over 130 pounds, and she's giving her skin every opportunity to bounce back, encouraging it with targeted exercise, heavy lifting, intelligent eating, taking a variety of daily supplements, and dry skin brushing.

All four women's stories, and Prim's story in particular, give us hope. Regardless of the current condition of our skin, our age and the amount of weight we have lost or still need to lose—losing weight, maintaining the loss, and firming loose skin is possible. They are an inspiration.

7

Summary: *What Now?*

Now that we've come to the end of the book, my head is spinning. Is yours?

There are so many options and possible treatments, and, if you're like me, you don't have unlimited time or a money tree in your yard. Of all the possibilities, how do we choose which ones to try first?

Below are what seem to be the best and most-effective suggestions from throughout the book. Concentrate on these before heading out to schedule plastic surgery. Give them a chance—let them work for you. You can get started on this list for well under $100. Given that skin-tightening surgery runs into the tens of thousands of dollars, that's not a bad deal at all.

I. **Go shopping for supplements, extracts, crèmes, lotions and oils.** The list in section three is comprehensive, they all are important, and a variety of them should be effective. After consulting with your doctor, you may want to try a few to start then incorporate the rest in time. Consider retinol, vitamins C and E, copper peptides, seaweed extract, hyaluronic acid and silica at first and the rest as time goes by. Be sure to take a good multivitamin daily and try to find one that incorporates as many of the substances listed in section three as is possible. You should be able to find these at your local pharmacy or online.

To save time and research when shopping online, you can visit this book's website at www.firmlooseskin.com or the book's Amazon.com store at http://astore.amazon.com/firlooski-20. And as you choose new supplements to incorporate, keep in mind what area you're targeting: reducing cellulite, building connective tissue, growing collagen, building muscle, or simply improving the appearance of your skin. All areas are important. Don't leave any out.

II. **Lift heavy weights.** Purchase *The New Rules of Lifting* or *The New Rules of Lifting for Women*. If you don't want to invest in joining a gym, you don't have to. Get a variety of free weights to use at home. Your local discount or sporting goods store is a great place to start.

III. **Buy a mini trampoline and jump on it.** Get one with a stability bar if you're uncoordinated. Be sure it's weight-tested to your specific body weight. They go up to 400 pounds, or more.

IV. **Do the facial exercises** in section four if you have loose skin on your face and neck.

V. **Buy a soft-bristled brush and perform dry skin brushing** every day before you shower, brushing gently towards your heart.

VI. **Drink your water!**

VII. **Cultivate and keep a good attitude**. Be positive and upbeat about your age, weight and skin condition. A negative attitude won't help. A positive attitude will help. Having a good attitude is key to losing weight, to aging with grace and it will help keep us motivated to do the things we need to do on a daily basis to help our skin tighten up.

VIII. **Consider sharing your story with others**. Visit the book's website at www.firmlooseskin.com to find out ways to connect, for updates and for the latest news on natural, effective skin-tightening treatments. Share what has worked and what hasn't so we can learn from each other. And, give it time. If you're looking for an instant solution, that's going to be plastic surgery. But if you're patient and willing to experiment, many of the suggestions in this book should help us both firm our loose skin.

Afterword:
Looking Like a Basset Hound,
Good or Bad?

In addition to writing and doing research, losing weight, and looking for ways to fight loose skin, my other passion is basset hounds and basset hound rescue.

Loose skin isn't particularly attractive on people but it's a hallmark of beauty on a basset hound. The American Kennel Club's official description of the breed standard for a basset hound specifies that the skin be "loose and elastic." Show-quality basset breeders breed for baggy skin among other distinctive characteristics like long ears, short legs and a powerful body.

I noticed this odd intersection of what I think is beautiful on a hound, and not particularly beautiful on myself, while researching the information that eventually coalesced into this book. And I thought that it would be fun to mention them in the book.

As with people, the older a basset hound gets, the more its skin sags and droops. My favorite animal rescue organization is a sanctuary for unwanted senior basset hounds that have nowhere else to go. Few people want to adopt older dogs, so House of Puddles in Frederick, Maryland takes in homeless senior bassets and provides them a loving home for the rest of their lives, saving them from being put to sleep because no one else wants them. If you visit www.houseofpuddles.org their sweet photos will make you smile.

House of Puddles is a 501(c)(3) nonprofit organization and all donations are tax deductible if you are moved to help them keep saving these droopy old basset hounds with their beautiful, saggy skin.

A portion of what you paid to purchase this book has been donated to basset hound rescue. My rescued basset hound

William and I thank you. And if you're interested in knowing more about how to help bassets in your area, visit The Daily Drool at http://www.dailydrool.com/rescue.html.

Finally, if basset hounds aren't your particular cup of tea, many other animals out there need your help. Please consider supporting your local animal shelter or rescue organization.

References and Resources for Further Reading

Abd El-Mohsen, M., Bayele, H., Kuhnle, G., Gibson, G., Debnam, E., Kaila Srai S., Rice-Evans, C., & Spencer, J.P. (2006, July). Distribution of [3H]trans-resveratrol in rat tissues following oral administration. *Br. J. Nutr.* 96(1), 62–70.

Abdominal Fat and What to Do About It. http://www.health.harvard.edu/newsweek/Abdominal-fat-and-what-to-do-about-it.htm

Abdulghani, A.A., Sherr, S., Shirin, S., Solodkina, G., Tapia, E.M., & Gottlieb, A.B. (1998). Effects of topical creams containing vitamin C, a copper-binding peptide cream and melatonin compared with tretinoin on the ultrastructure of normal skin - A pilot clinical, histologic, and ultrastructural study. *Disease Manag Clin Outcomes.* 1:136-141.

Abdulghani, A.A., Shirin, S., Morales-Tapio, A., Sherr, G., Solodkina, M., Roberson, & Gottlieb, A.B. (1998). Studies of the effects of topical vitamin C, a copper binding cream and melatonin cream as compared with tretinoin on the ultrastructure of the skin, *J. Invest. Dematol.* 110(4), 686.

Abelson, B.J. & Abelson, K. (Retrieved 2012). The effects of nutrition on traumatic injury to connective tissue. *Kinetic Health.* http://www.drabelson.com/trauma.html

Abelson, P. (1999, March). A Potential Phosphate Crisis. *Science.* 283 (5410): 2015.

Adams, A. (2011, August 7). What Are the Health Benefits of Phytessence Wakame? http://www.livestrong.com/article/470047-what-are-the-health-benefits-of-phytessence-wakame/

Adkins, J. (Retrieved 2012). 5 Vitamins for Healthy Skin. http://skincare.about.com/od/skin101/tp/VitaminsinHealthySkin.htm

Aesculus hippocastanum (Horse chestnut). (2009). *Alternative Medicine Review.* (14)3.

Ageless. (Retrieved 2012). Neck and Throat Facial Exercises. http://www.ageless.co.za/facialneck.htm

Ageless. (Retrieved 2012). Lips and Cheeks Facial Exercises. http://www.ageless.co.za/faciallip.htm

Ageless. (Retrieved 2012). Eyes and Forehead Facial Exercises. http://www.ageless.co.za/facialeye.htm

Aggarwal, B.B. & Shishodia, S. (2006). Molecular targets of dietary agents for prevention and therapy of cancer. *Biochem. Pharmacol.* 71(10): 1397–421.

Ahmed, M.R., Basha, S.H., Gopinath, D., Muthusamy, R., & Jayakumar, R. (2005). Initial upregulation of growth factors and inflammatory mediators during nerve regeneration in the presence of cell adhesive peptide-incorporated collagen tubes. *J. Peripher. Nerv. Syst.* 10,1:17-30.

Ahn, D., Putt, D., Kresty, L., Stoner, G.D., Fromm, D., & Hollenberg, P.F. (1996). The effects of dietary ellagic acid on rat hepatic and esophageal mucosal cytochromes P450 and phase II enzymes. *Carcinogenesis.* 17:821-828.

AKC Meet the Breeds: Get to Know the Basset Hound. (Retrieved 2012). http://www.akc.org/breeds/basset_hound/index.cfm

Akiba, S., Matsugo, S., Packer, L., & Konishi, T. (1998). Assay of protein-bound lipoic acid in tissues by a new enzymatic method. *Analytical Biochemistry.* 258(2): 299–304.

Alanine. (Retrieved 2012). http://www.evitamins.com/encyclopedia/assets/nutritional-supplement/alanine/side-effects

Albanes, D. (1999). Beta-carotene and lung cancer: a case study. *Am J Clin Nutr* 69(6): 1345S–50S.

Alcaín, F.J. & Villalba, J.M. (April 2009). Sirtuin activators. *Expert Opin Ther Pat.* 19(4): 403–14.

Aleccia, J. (2008, April 22). Longevity quest moves slowly from lab to life. *MSNBC.* http://www.msnbc.msn.com/id/23359040/

Alexiades-Armenakas, M., Dover, J.S. & Arndt, K.A. (2008, September). Unipolar radiofrequency treatment to improve the appearance of cellulite. *J. Cosmet. Laser Ther.* 10(3): 148-53.

Al-Hadithy, H., Isenberg, D.A., Addison, I.E., Goldstone, A.H. & Snaith, M.L. (1982). Neutrophil function in systemic lupus erythematosus and other collagen diseases. *Ann Rheum Dis.* 41(1): 33–38.

All About Amino Acids: Alanine. (Retrieved 2012). http://www.vitalhealthzone.com/nutrition/amino-acids/alanine.html

Alpha Lipoic Acid. (Retrieved 2012). http://www.vitaminstuff.com/alpha-lipoic-acid.html

Alpha Lipoic Acid Side Effects. (Retrieved 2012). http://www.whathealth.com/alphalipoicacid/sideeffects.html

Alvarez-Lario, B. & Macarron-Vicente, J. (2010). Uric acid and evolution. *Rheumatology.* 49(11): 2010–5.

American Academy of Dermatology. (2007, August 5). New Technologies Tighten Skin From Head To Toe Without Surgery. *ScienceDaily.* http://www.sciencedaily.com/releases/2007/08/070803145744.htm

American Academy of Dermatology. (2010, August). Cosmetic Procedures: Fillers. http://www.skincarephysicians.com/agingskinnet/fillers.html

American Chemical Society. (2009, June 17). New Evidence That Vinegar May Be Natural Fat Fighter. http://portal.acs.org/portal/acs/corg/content?_nfpb=true&_pageLabel=PP_ARTICLEMAIN&node_id=223&content_id=CNBP_022291&use_sec=true&sec_url_var=region1&__uuid=#P102_8297

American Medical Association. (1987, April 24). Burn treatment for the unburned. *Journal of the American Medical Association.* 257(16), 2207-2208.

Ames, B., Cathcart, R., Schwiers, E. & Hochstein, P. (1981). Uric acid provides an antioxidant defense in humans against oxidant- and radical-caused aging and cancer: a hypothesis. *Proc Natl Acad Sci USA.* 78 (11): 6858–62. http://www.ncbi.nlm.nih.gov/pmc/articles/PMC349151/

Amino Acids and Their Significance for Anti-Aging. (Retrieved 2012). http://www.aminoacid-studies.com/areas-of-use/anti-aging.html

Amorini, A.M., Petzold, A., Tavazzi, B., Eikelenboom, J., Keir, G., Belli, A., Giovannoni, G., Di Pietro, V. *et al.* (2009). Increase of uric acid and purine compounds in biological fluids of multiple sclerosis patients. *Clinical Biochemistry.* 42(10–11): 1001–6.

Anderson, J. (2008). *Homemade Supplement Secrets.* http://www.buildmusclefastreviews.com/bodybuilding-supplements/homemade-supplement-secrets-review/

Anekonda, T.S. (2006, September). Resveratrol--a boon for treating Alzheimer's disease? *Brain Res Rev.* 52(2): 316–26.

Ansari, K.A., Vavia, P.R., Trotta, F. & Cavalli, R. (2011, March). Cyclodextrin-based nanosponges for delivery of resveratrol: in vitro characterisation, stability, cytotoxicity and permeation study. *AAPS PharmSciTech.* 12(1): 279–86. http://www.ncbi.nlm.nih.gov/pmc/articles/PMC3066340/

Antioxidant may prevent alcohol-induced liver disease. (2011, May 2). e! Science News. http://esciencenews.com/articles/2011/05/02/antioxidant.may.prevent.alcohol.induced.liver.disease?utm_source=feedburner&utm_medium=feed&utm_campaign=Feed%3A+eScienceNews%2Fpopular+%28e!+Science+News+-+Popular%29

Antioxidants and Cancer Prevention: Fact Sheet. (2007, March 4). National Cancer Institute. http://www.cancer.gov/cancertopics/factsheet/prevention/antioxidants

Are Detox Diets Safe? (Retrieved 2012). http://kidshealth.org/PageManager.jsp?dn=American_Academy_of_Family_Physicians&lic=44&cat_id=20131&article_set=21997&ps=204

Armstrong, G.A. & Hearst, J.E. (1996). Carotenoids 2: Genetics and molecular biology of carotenoid pigment biosynthesis. *FASEB J.* 10(2): 228–37.

Arnér, E. & Holmgren, A. (2000). Physiological functions of thioredoxin and thioredoxin reductase. *Eur J Biochem,* 267(20): 6102–9.

Arnold, G. (2011, March 16). Quercetin reduces markers of oxidative stress and inflammation. *Clinical Nutrition.* http://www.now-university.com/Library/HealthConcerns/AllergyImmuneSystem/082276.htm

Arroyo, A., Navarro, F., Navas, P. & Villalba, J.M. (1998). Ubiquinol regeneration by plasma membrane ubiquinone reductase. *Protoplasma* 205 (1-4): 107–113.

Asensi, M., Medina, I., Ortega, A., Carretero, J., Baño, M.C., Obrador, E. & Estrela, J.M. (2002, August). Inhibition of cancer growth by resveratrol is related to its low bioavailability. *Free Radic. Biol. Med.* 33(3): 387–98.

Association for Research and Enlightenment. (Retrieved 2012). Cayce Health Database: Castor Oil Packs. http://www.edgarcayce.org/are/holistic_health/data/thcast1.html

Athar, M., Back, J.H., Tang, X., Kim, K.H., Kopelovich, L., Bickers, D.R. & Kim, A.L. (2007, November). Resveratrol: a review of preclinical studies for human cancer prevention. *Toxicol. Appl. Pharmacol.* 224(3): 274–83. http://www.ncbi.nlm.nih.gov/pmc/articles/PMC2083123/

Atkinson, J., Epand, R.F. & Epand, R.M. (2008). Tocopherols and tocotrienols in membranes: A critical review. *Free Radical Biology and Medicine.* 44(5): 739–64.

Aviram, M. (2000). Review of human studies on oxidative damage and antioxidant protection related to cardiovascular diseases. *Free Radic Res.* 33 Suppl: S85–97.

Aviram, M., Rosenblat, M., Gaitini, D. *et al.* (2004, June). Pomegranate juice consumption for 3 years by patients with carotid artery stenosis reduces common carotid intima-media thickness, blood pressure and LDL oxidation. *Clin Nutr.* 23(3): 423–33.

Azam, S., Hadi, N., Khan, N.U. & Hadi, S.M. (2003, September). Antioxidant and prooxidant properties of caffeine, theobromine and xanthine. *Medi Sci Monit.* 9(9): BR325-30. http://www.ncbi.nlm.nih.gov/pubmed/12960921

Aziz, M.H., Nihal, M., Fu, V.X., Jarrard, D.F. & Ahmad, N. (2006, May). Resveratrol-caused apoptosis of human prostate carcinoma LNCaP cells is mediated via modulation of phosphatidylinositol 3'-kinase/Akt pathway and Bcl-2 family proteins. *Mol. Cancer Ther.* 5 (5): 1335–41.

Azzi, A. (2007). Molecular mechanism of α-tocopherol action. *Free Radical Biology and Medicine.* 43(1): 16–21.

Babu, T.D., Kuttan, G. & Padikkala, J. (1995). Cytotoxic and anti-tumour properties of certain taxa of Umbelliferae with special reference to Centella asiatica (L.) Urban. *J Ethnopharmacol.* 48:53-7.

Bachmanov, A.A., Reed, D.R., Tordoff, M.G., Price, R.A. & Beauchamp, G.K. (2001, March). Nutrient preference and diet-induced adiposity in C57BL/6ByJ and 129P3/J mice. *Physiology & Behavior.* 72(31–9384): 603–613.

Bae, J.Y., Choi, J.S., Kang, S.W., Lee, Y.J., Park, J. & Kang, Y.H. (2010, August). Dietary compound ellagic acid alleviates skin wrinkle and inflammation induced by UV-B irradiation. *Exp Dermatol.* 19(8):e182-90.

Balch, P.A. (2010). *Prescription for Nutritional Healing, Fifth Edition: A Practical A-to-Z Reference to Drug-Free Remedies Using Vitamins, Minerals, Herbs & Food Supplements.* Avery.

Bannister, J., Bannister, W. & Rotilio, G. (1987). Aspects of the structure, function, and applications of superoxide dismutase. *CRC Crit Rev Biochem.* 22(2): 111–80.

Baral, J. (2001, July 19). What Are Free Radicals? http://www.ivillage.com/what-are-free-radicals-skin-expert-dr-jim-baral-ivillage-beauty-skin-clinic/5-a-147111

Barger, J.L., Kayo, T., Vann, J.M., Arias, E.B., Wang, J., Hacker, T.A., Wang, Y., Raederstorff, D., Morrow, J.D., Leeuwenburgh, C., Allison, D.B., Saupe, K.W., Cartee, G.D., Weindruch, R. & Prolla, T.A. (2008). Tomé, D., ed. A low dose of dietary resveratrol partially mimics caloric restriction and retards aging parameters in mice. *PLoS ONE.* 3(6): e2264. http://www.ncbi.nlm.nih.gov/pmc/articles/PMC2386967/

Barolet, D. (2008). Light-emitting diodes (LEDs) in dermatology. *Seminars in Cutaneous Medicine and Surgery.* 27:227-238. http://www.babyquasar.com/PDF/LEDs_in_dermatology.pdf

Barrager, E., Veltmann, J.R., Schauss, A.G. & Schiller, R.N. (2002, April). A multi-centered, open label trial on the safety and efficacy of methylsulfonylmethane in the treatment of seasonal allergic rhinitis. *Journal of Alternative and Complementary Medicine.* 8(2): 167-173. http://www.ncbi.nlm.nih.gov/pubmed/12006124

Barros, M.H., Bandy, B., Tahara, E.B. & Kowaltowski, A.J. (2004). Higher respiratory activity decreases mitochondrial reactive oxygen release and increases life span in Saccharomyces cerevisiae. *J. Biol. Chem.* 279 (48): 49883–8.

Bass, T.M., Weinkove, D., Houthoofd, K., Gems, D. & Partridge, L. (October 2007). Effects of resveratrol on lifespan in Drosophila melanogaster and Caenorhabditis elegans. *Mech. Ageing Dev.* 128 (10): 546–52.

Basu, A. & Imrhan, V. (2007). Tomatoes versus lycopene in oxidative stress and carcinogenesis: conclusions from clinical trials. *Eur J Clin Nutr,* 61(3): 295–303.

Bates, C. & Yinka, T. (2009, September 25). Tone and tighten with a rebounding six week workout. *Daily Mail.* http://www.dailymail.co.uk/health/article-1213310/Tone-Tighten-Rebounding-Six-Week-Workout.html

Battino, M., Ferri, E., Gorini, A., *et al.* (1990). Natural distribution and occurrence of coenzyme Q homologues. *Membr Biochem.* 9(3): 179–90.

Bauer, J. (2012). Eat Your Way to Beautiful Skin. http://www.joybauer.com/healthy-living/food-for-beautiful-skin.aspx

Baumann, L. (2007, November 30). Skin Type Solutions: Supplements and Skin Care: An A to Z Guide. http://www.skintypesolutions.com/newsletters/178-supplements-and-skin-care-an-a-to-z-guide

Baur, J.A., Pearson, K.J., Price, N.L., Jamieson, H.A., Lerin, C., Kalra, A., Prabhu, V.V., Allard, J.S., Lopez-Lluch, G., Lewis, K., Pistell, P.J., Poosala, S., Becker, K.G., Boss, O., Gwinn, D., Wang, M., Ramaswamy, S., Fishbein, K.W., Spencer, R.G., Lakatta, E.G., Le Couteur, D., Shaw, R.J., Navas, P., Puigserver, P., Ingram, D.K., de Cabo, R. & Sinclair, D.A. (2006, November). Resveratrol improves health and survival of mice on a high-calorie diet. *Nature.* 444(7117): 337–42.

Baur, J.A. & Sinclair, D.A. (2006, June). Therapeutic potential of resveratrol: the in vivo evidence. *Nat Rev Drug Discov.* 5(6): 493–506.

Becker, B. (1993). Towards the physiological function of uric acid. *Free Radical Biology and Medicine.* 14(6): 615–31.

Beecher, G. (2003). Overview of dietary flavonoids: nomenclature, occurrence and intake. *J Nutr.* 133(10): 3248S–3254S. http://jn.nutrition.org/content/133/10/3248S.full

Beher, D., Wu, J., Cumine, S., Kim, K.W., Lu, S.C., Atangan, L. & Wang, M. (2009, December). Resveratrol is not a direct activator of SIRT1 enzyme activity. *Chem Biol Drug Des.* 74(6): 619–24.

Belcaro, G.V., Rulo, A. & Grimaldi, R. (1990). Capillary filtration and ankle edema in patients with venous hypertension treated with TTFCA. *Angiology.* 41:12-8.

Bell, S. (2010, July 21). Neck Skin Tightening Exercises. http://www.livestrong.com/article/180912-neck-skin-tightening-exercises/

Benitez, D.A., Pozo-Guisado, E., Alvarez-Barrientos, A., Fernandez-Salguero, P.M. & Castellón, E.A. (2007). Mechanisms involved in resveratrol-induced apoptosis and cell cycle arrest in prostate cancer-derived cell lines. *J. Androl.* 28(2): 282–93.

Bennett, A. (2011, June 14). Collagen Supplements for Weight Loss. http://www.livestrong.com/article/254415-collagen-supplements-for-weight-loss/#ixzz26eWT8q4K

Bennett, A. (2011, August 11). What Does the Amino Acid L-Ornithine Do? http://www.livestrong.com/article/22017-amino-acid-l-ornithine/

Benzie, I. (2003). Evolution of dietary antioxidants. *Comparative Biochemistry and Physiology.* 136(1): 113–26.

Berry, Y. (Retrieved 2012). Alternative Cures: Discover Natural Solutions for Health & Beauty. http://blog.greathomeremedies.com/

Bertelli, A.A., Gozzini, A., Stradi, R., Stella, S. & Bertelli, A. (1998). Stability of resveratrol over time and in the various stages of grape transformation. *Drugs Exp Clin Res* 24 (4): 207–11.

Berti, F., Omini, C. & Longiave, D. (1977, August). The mode of action of aescin and the release of prostaglandins. *Prostaglandins.* 14(2): 241–249.

Bhat, K.P., Lantvit, D., Christov, K., Mehta, R.G., Moon, R.C. & Pezzuto, J.M. (2001, October). Estrogenic and antiestrogenic properties of resveratrol in mammary tumor models. *Cancer Res.* 61(20): 7456–63.

Bhattacharya, A., McCutcheon, E. P., Shvartz, E. & Greenleaf, J. E. (1980, November 1). Body acceleration and O2 uptake in humans during running and jumping. *Journal of Applied Physiology*, 49, 5, 881-887.

Bioflavonoids Consumer Information. (Retrieved 2012). http://www.drugs.com/mtm/bioflavonoids.html

Bishop, J.B., Phillips, L.G., Mustoe, T.A., VanderZee, A.J., Wiersema, L., Roach, D.E., Heggers, J.P., Hill Jr, D.P. *et al.* (1992, August). A prospective randomized evaluator-blinded trial of two potential wound healing agents for the treatment of venous stasis ulcers. *J Vasc Surg.* 16(2): 251–257.

Bjelakovic, G., Nagorni, A., Nikolova, D., Simonetti, R., Bjelakovic, M. & Gluud, C. (2006). Meta-analysis: antioxidant supplements for primary and secondary prevention of colorectal adenoma. *Aliment. Pharmacol. Ther.* 24(2): 281–91.

Bjelakovic, G., Nikolova, D., Gluud, L.L., Simonetti, R.G. & Gluud, C. (2007). Mortality in randomized trials of antioxidant supplements for primary and secondary prevention: systematic review and meta-analysis. *JAMA.* 297(8): 842–57. jama.jamanetwork.com/article.aspx? articleid=205797

Bjelakovic, G., Nikolova, D., Gluud, L.L., Simonetti, R.G. & Gluud, C. (2008). Bjelakovic, G., ed. Antioxidant supplements for prevention of mortality in healthy participants and patients with various diseases. *Cochrane Database of Systematic Reviews.* (2)CD007176.

Blank, C. (2010, July 29). The Side Effects of Cocoa Butter. http://www.livestrong.com/article/188407-the-side-effects-of-cocoa-butter/

Bleys, J., Miller, E., Pastor-Barriuso, R., Appel, L. & Guallar, E. (2006). Vitamin-mineral supplementation and the progression of atherosclerosis: a meta-analysis of randomized controlled trials. *Am. J. Clin. Nutr.* 84(4): 880–7.

Block, K.I., Koch, A.C., Mead, M.N., Tothy, P.K., Newman, R.A. & Gyllenhaal, C. (2008). Impact of antioxidant supplementation on chemotherapeutic toxicity: a systematic review of the evidence from randomized controlled trials. *Int. J. Cancer.* 123(6): 1227–39.

Blow, N. (2009). Cell culture: building a better matrix. *Nature Methods* 6 (8): 619–622.

Boileau, T.W., Liao, Z., Kim, S. *et al.* (2003). Prostate carcinogenesis in N-methyl-Nitrosourea (NMU)-testosterone-treated rats fed tomato powder, lycopene, or energy-restricted diets. *J Natl Cancer Inst.* 95:1578-1586.

Bond, A.B. (Retrieved 2012). Beautiful Skin Tip: Apple Cider Vinegar. http://www.care2.com/greenliving/apple-cider-vinegar-skin-tip.html

Bond, O. (2011, July 15). What Is the Benefit of Collagen Vitamins? http://www.livestrong.com/article/493387-what-is-the-benefit-of-collagen-vitamins/#ixzz26ZosmHDu

Bosse, J.P., Papillon, J., Frenette, G. *et al.* (1979). Clinical study of a new antikeloid agent. *Ann Plast Surg.* 3:13,21.

Bowers, J.L., Tyulmenkov, V.V., Jernigan, S.C. & Klinge, C.M. (2000, October). Resveratrol acts as a mixed agonist/antagonist for estrogen receptors alpha and beta. *Endocrinology* . 141(10): 3657–67.

Bowtell, J.L., Gelly, K., Jackman, M.L., Patel, A., Simeoni, M. & Rennie, M.J. (1999). Effect of oral glutamine on whole body carbohydrate storage during recovery from exhaustive exercise. *Journal of Applied Physiology.* 86(6): 1770-1777.

Bradwejn, J., Zhou Y., Koszycki, D. & Shlik, J. (2000). A double-blind, placebo-controlled study on the effects of Gotu Kola (Centella asiatica) on acoustic startle response in healthy subjects. *J Clin Psychopharmacol.* 20:680-4.

Bråkenhielm, E., Cao, R. & Cao, Y. (2001, August). Suppression of angiogenesis, tumor growth, and wound healing by resveratrol, a natural compound in red wine and grapes. *FASEB J.* 15(10): 1798–800.

Breitkreutz, D., Mirancea, N. & Nischt, R. (2009). Basement membranes in skin: Unique matrix structures with diverse functions? *Histochemistry and cell biology* . 132(1): 1–10.

Brien, S., Prescott, P., Bashir, N., Lewith, H. & Lewith, G. (November 2008). Systematic review of the nutritional supplements dimethyl sulfoxide (DMSO) and methylsulfonylmethane (MSM) in the treatment of osteoarthritis. *Osteoarthritis Cartilage,* 16(11), 1277-1288.

Brigelius-Flohé, R. (1999). Tissue-specific functions of individual gluta-thione peroxidases. *Free Radic Biol Med.* 27(9–10): 951–65.

Brigelius-Flohé, R. & Davies, K.J.A. (2007). Is vitamin E an antioxidant, a regulator of signal transduction and gene expression, or a 'junk' food? Comments on the two accompanying papers: 'Molecular mechanism of α-tocopherol action' by A. Azzi and 'Vitamin E, antioxidant and nothing more' by M. Traber and J. Atkinson. *Free Radical Biology and Medicine* 43(1): 2–3.

Brigelius-Flohé, R. & Traber, M.G. (1999). Vitamin E: Function and metabolism. *The FASEB Journal.* 13(10): 1145–55. http://www.fasebj.org/content/13/10/1145.long

Brinkhaus, B., Lindner, M., Schuppan, D. & Hahn, E.G. (2000). Chemical, pharmacological and clinical profile of the east Asian medical plant Centella asiatica. *Phytomedicine.* 7:427-48.

Brito, P.M., Devillard, R., Nègre-Salvayre, A., Almeida, L.M., Dinis, T.C., Salvayre, R. & Augé, N. (2009, July). Resveratrol inhibits the mTOR mitogenic signaling evoked by oxidized LDL in smooth muscle cells. *Atherosclerosis.* 205(1): 126–34.

Britton, G., Liaaen-Jensen, S. & Pfander, H. (1996). *Carotenoids: Synthesis (Carotenoids).* Boston: Birkhauser.

Brodie, D., Moscrip, V. & Hutcheon, R. (1998). Body Composition Measurement: A Review of Hydrodensitometry, Anthropometry, and Impedance Methods. *Nutrition.* 14(3): 296–310.

Brown, G.L. (1995, November). Enhancement of wound healing by biosynthetic growth factors. U.S. Army Medical Research and Materiel Command. Fort Detrick, MD.

Brown, N. (2010, July 20). Natural Ways to Remove Cellulite. http://www.livestrong.com/article/179423-natural-ways-to-remove-cellulite/

Bucci, L.R. (1995). *Nutrition Applied to Injury Rehabilitation and Sports Medicine.* Boca Raton: CRC Press.

Buehler, M.J. (2006). Nature designs tough collagen: Explaining the nano-structure of collagen fibrils. *PNAS.* 103(33): 12285–12290.

Campbell, J.K., Canene-Adams, K., Lindshield, B.L., Boileau, T.W., Clinton, S.K. & Erdman, Jr., J.W. (2004). Tomato phytochemicals and prostate cancer risk. *J Nutr.* 134:3486S-3492S.

Canapp, Jr., S.O., Farese, J.P., Schultz, G.S., Gowda, S., Ishak, A.M., Swaim, S.F., Vangilder, J., Lee-Ambrose, L. & Martin, F.G. (2003). The effect of topical tripeptide-copper complex on healing of ischemic open wounds. *Vet Surg.* 32(6):515-23.

Cangul, I.T., Gul, N.Y., Topal, A. & Yilmaz, R. (2006). Evaluation of the effects of topical tripeptide-copper complex and zinc oxide on open-wound healing in rabbits. *Vet Dermatol.* 17(6):417-23.

Cao, G., Alessio, H. & Cutler, R. (1993). Oxygen-radical absorbance capacity assay for antioxidants. *Free Radic Biol Med.* 14(3): 303–11.

Cao, Y., Fu, Z.D., Wang, F., Liu, H.Y. & Han, R. (2005, June). Anti-angiogenic activity of resveratrol, a natural compound from medicinal plants. *J Asian Nat Prod Res.* 7(3): 205–13.

Carr, A. & Frei, B. (1999). Does vitamin C act as a pro-oxidant under physiological conditions? *FASEB J.* 13(9): 1007–24. www.fasebj.org/ content/13/9/1007.full

Carter, A.E. (1979). Rebound exercise is the most efficient, effective form of exercise yet devised by man. *The Miracles of Rebound Exercise, The National institute of Reboundology and Health, Inc.*: Edmonds, Washington. http://www.rebound-aerobics.com/NASA_rebounder_report2.htm

Casco, K. (2010, November 25). Side Effects of Vitamin E Skin Oil. http://www.livestrong.com/article/317819-side-effects-of-vitamin-e-skin-oil/

Catherine. (2012, September 24). Personal communication.

Caution urged with resveratrol. (2006, November 30). *United Press International.* http://www.upi.com/Science_News/2006/11/30/Caution-urged-with-resveratrol/UPI-95041164906073/

Cellulite. (Retrieved 2012). http://www.greathomeremedies.com/cellulite.html

Cellulite Guide. (Retrieved 2012). http://celluliteguide.org/

Cellulitis. (2011, May 13). http://www.ncbi.nlm.nih.gov/pubmedhealth/PMH0001858/

Cesarone, M.R., Belcaro, G., De Sanctis, M.T. et al. (2001). Effects of the total triterpenic fraction of Centella asiatica in venous hypertensive microangiopathy: a prospective, placebo-controlled, randomized trial. *Angiology.* 52 Suppl 2:S15-18.

Chaudiere, J. & Ferrari-Iliou, R. (1999). Intracellular antioxidants: From chemical to biochemical mechanisms. *Food and Chemical Toxicology.* 37(9–10): 949–62.

Chelikani, P., Fita, I. & Loewen, P. (2004). Diversity of structures and properties among catalases. *Cell Mol Life Sci.* 61(2): 192–208.

Chemists Kill Cancer Cells With Light-activated Molecules. (2007, August 9). ScienceDaily. http://www.sciencedaily.com/releases/2007/08/070808132019.htm

Chen, C., Sander, J.E. & Dale, N.M. (2003). The effect of dietary lysine deficiency on the immune response to Newcastle disease vaccination in chickens. *Avian Dis.* 47(4): 1346–51.

Chen, C.K. & Pace-Asciak, C.R. (1996, March). Vasorelaxing activity of resveratrol and quercetin in isolated rat aorta. *Gen. Pharmacol.* 27(2): 363–6.

Cheng, C.L. & Koo, M.W.L. (2000). Effects of Centella asiatica on ethanol induced gastric mucosal lesions in rats. *Life Sci.* 67:2647-53.

Cherkin, A. & Exkardt, M.J. (1977, January). Effects of dimethyl-aminoethanol upon life-span and behavior of aged Japanese quail. *J Gerontol.* 32(1): 38–45. http://geronj.oxfordjournals.org/content/32/ 1/38.long

Cherubini, A., Vigna, G., Zuliani, G., Ruggiero, C., Senin, U. & Fellin, R. (2005). Role of antioxidants in atherosclerosis: epidemiological and clinical update. *Curr Pharm Des.* 11(16): 2017–32.

Chun, Y.J., Kim, M.Y. & Guengerich, F.P. (1999, August). Resveratrol is a selective human cytochrome P450 1A1 inhibitor. *Biochem. Biophys. Res. Commun.* 262(1): 20–4.

Cichewicz, R.H., Kouzi, S.A. & Hamann, M.T. (2000). Dimerization of resveratrol by the grapevine pathogen Botrytis cinerea. *Journal of Natural Products* 63(1): 29–33.

Clark, P.E., Hall, M.C., Borden, Jr., L.S. *et al.* (2006). Phase I-II prospective dose-escalating trial of lycopene in patients with biochemical relapse of prostate cancer after definitive local therapy. *Urology.* 67:1257-1261.

Clark, G., Parker, E., Schaad, J. & Warren, W. J. (1935). New measurements of previously unknown large interplanar spacings in natural materials. *J. Amer. Chem. Soc.* 57(8): 1509.

Clarke, N. (2011, October 25). B-12 for Lymph Nodes. http://www.livestrong.com/article/549510-b-12-for-lymph-nodes/#ixzz261D6vhYL

Clément, K, Vaisse, C., Lahlou, N., Cabrol, S., Pelloux, V., Cassuto, D., Gourmelen, M., Dina, C., Chambaz, J., Lacorte, J.M., Basdevant, A., Bougnères, P., Lebouc, Y., Froguel, P. & Guy-Grand, B. (1998, March 26). A mutation in the human leptin receptor gene causes obesity and pituitary dysfunction. *Nature.* 392(6674):398-401.

Cleren, C., Yang, L., Lorenzo, B. *et al.* (2008, March). Therapeutic effects of coenzyme Q10 (CoQ10) and reduced CoQ10 in the MPTP model of Parkinsonism. *J. Neurochem.* 104(6): 1613–21.

Cleveland Clinic. (2011, March 24). Understanding the Ingredients in Skin Care Products. http://my.clevelandclinic.org/healthy_living/skin_care/hic_understanding_the_ingredients_in_skin_care_products.aspx

Close, G., Ashton, T., Cable, T., Doran, D., Holloway, C., McArdle, F. & MacLaren, D. (2006). Ascorbic acid supplementation does not attenuate post-exercise muscle soreness following muscle-damaging exercise but may delay the recovery process. *Br J Nutr.* 95(5): 976–81.

Coker, R.H., Williams, R., Kortebein, P., Sullivan, D. & Evans, W. (2009). Influence of exercise intensity on abdominal fat and adiponectin in elderly adults. *Metabolic Syndrome and Related Disorders.* 7(4): 363–368.

Collagen and Other Injectable Fillers. (Retrieved 2012). http://www.webmd.com/healthy-beauty/collagen-injections

Complete Methylsulfonylmethane (MSM) Information. (Retrieved 2012). http://www.drugs.com/npp/methylsulfonylmethane-msm.html

Conato *et al.* (2001). Copper complexes of glycyl-histidyl-lysine and two of its synthetic analogues: chemical behaviour and biological activity. *Biochim Biophys Acta.* 3, 1526(2):199-210.

Connective Tissue. (Retrieved 2012). http://www.courseweb.uottawa.ca/medicine-histology/English/SS_BasicTissues/Connective_Tissue.htm

Cook, N.R., Albert, C.M. & Gaziano, J.M. (2007). A randomized factorial trial of vitamins C and E and beta carotene in the secondary prevention of cardiovascular events in women: results from the Women's Antioxidant Cardiovascular Study.

Arch. Intern. Med. 167(15): 1610–8. http://www.ncbi.nlm.nih.gov/pmc/articles/PMC2034519/

Corder, R., Mullen, W., Khan, N.Q., Marks, S.C., Wood, E.G., Carrier, M.J. & Crozier, A. (2006, November). Oenology: red wine procyanidins and vascular health. *Nature.* 444(7119): 566.

Cosmetic Surgery Unnecessary With New Technology to Tighten Skin: Skin-Tightening Technology Can Treat Sagging Skin Without Surgery. (2007, August 6). http://voices.yahoo.com/cosmetic-surgery-unnecessary-technology-to-480088.html?cat=69

Coulter, I., Hardy, M., Morton, S., Hilton, L., Tu, W., Valentine, D. & Shekelle, P. (2006). Antioxidants vitamin C and vitamin E for the prevention and treatment of cancer. *Journal of General Internal Medicine: Official Journal of the Society for Research and Education in Primary Care Internal Medicine.* 21(7): 735–44. http://www.ncbi.nlm.nih.gov/pmc/articles/PMC1924689/

Cousin, P.J. (2001). *Anti-Wrinkle Treatments for Perfect Skin.* Storey Books.

Coyne, J.A. (1999, October 10). The Truth Is Way Out There. *The New York Times.* http://www.nytimes.com/1999/10/10/books/the-truth-is-way-out-there.html

Creatine Information Page. (Retrieved 2012). http://www.anyvitamins.com/creatine-info.htm

Creissen, G., Broadbent, P., Stevens, R., Wellburn, A. & Mullineaux, P. (1996). Manipulation of glutathione metabolism in transgenic plants. *Biochem Soc Trans.* 24(2): 465–9.

Cullen, J.J., Weydert, C., Hinkhouse, M.M., Ritchie, J., Domann, F.E., Spitz, D. & Oberley, L.W. (2003, March). The role of manganese superoxide dismutase in the growth of pancreatic adenocarcinoma. *Cancer Res.* 63(6): 1297–303.

Cúneo, F., Costa-Paiva, L., Pinto-Neto, A.M., Morais, S.S. & Amaya-Farfan, J. (2010, March). Effect of dietary supplementation with collagen hydrolysates on bone metabolism of postmenopausal women with low mineral density. *Maturitas.* 65(3):253-7.

Curran, M.E., Atkinson, D.L., Ewart, A.K., Morris, C.A., Leppert, M.F. & Keating, M.T. (1993, April). The elastin gene is disrupted by a translocation associated with supravalvular aortic stenosis. *Cell.* 73(1): 159–68.

Cypess, A.M., Lehman, S., Williams, G., Tal, I., Rodman, D., Goldfine, A.B., Kuo, F.C., Palmer, E.L. *et al.* (2009). Identification and importance of brown adipose tissue in adult humans. *The New England Journal of Medicine.* 360(15): 1509–17.

Cystine [sp] Information Page. (Retrieved 2012). http://www.anyvitamins.com/cystine-info.htm

Dangers of Alpha Hydroxy Acids. (2011, June 14). http://www.livestrong.com/article/369298-dangers-of-alpha-hydroxy-acids/

Daniells, S. (2009, June 18). Could Vinegar Be Natural Fat Fighter? http://www.nutraingredients.com/Research/Could-vinegar-be-natural-fat-fighter

Das, D.K. & Maulik, N. (2006, February). Resveratrol in cardioprotection: a therapeutic promise of alternative medicine. *Mol. Interv.* 6(1): 36–47.

Deanol. (Retrieved 2012). http://www.webmd.com/vitamins-supplements/ingredientmono-524-DEANOL.aspx?activeIngredientId=524&activeIngredientName=DEANOL

Debunking the Myths of Colon Cleansing. (2010). http://cchealth.clevelandclinic.org/also-issue/debunking-myths-colon-cleansing

Dekkers, J., van Doornen, L. & Kemper, H. (1996). The role of antioxidant vitamins and enzymes in the prevention of exercise-induced muscle damage. *Sports Med.* 21(3): 213–38.

Del Carlo, M., Sacchetti, G., Di Mattia, C., Compagnone, D., Mastrocola, D., Liberatore, L. & Cichelli, A. (2004). Contribution of the phenolic fraction to the antioxidant activity and oxidative stability of olive oil. *J Agric Food Chem.* 52(13): 4072–9.

del Río, L., Sandalio, L., Palma, J., Bueno, P. & Corpas, F. (1992). Metabolism of oxygen radicals in peroxisomes and cellular implications. *Free Radic Biol Med.* 13(5): 557–80.

Demmig-Adams, B. & Adams, W.W., 3rd. (2002). Antioxidants in photosynthesis and human nutrition. *Science.* 298(5601): 2149–53.

Denese, A. (2005). *Dr. Denese's Secrets for Ageless Skin.* New York: Berkeley Publishing Group.

Deng, J.Y., Hsieh, P.S., Huang, J.P., Lu, L.S. & Hung, L.M. (2008, July). Activation of estrogen receptor is crucial for resveratrol-stimulating muscular glucose uptake via both insulin-dependent and -independent pathways. *Diabetes.* 57 (7): 1814–23. http://www.ncbi.nlm.nih.gov/ pmc/articles/PMC2453636/

Derby, C.A., Zilber, S., Brambilla, D., Morales, K.H. & McKinlay, J.B. (2006). Body mass index, waist circumference and waist to hip ratio and change in sex steroid hormones: the Massachusetts Male Ageing Study. *Clin Endocrinol (Oxf).* 65(1): 125-131.

Di Lullo, G.A. (2002). Mapping the Ligand-binding sites and disease-associated mutations on the most abundant protein in the human, type I collagen. *Journal of Biological Chemistry.* 277(6): 4223–31.

Di Mascio, P., Kaiser, S. & Sies, H. (1989). Lycopene as the most efficient biological carotenoid singlet oxygen quencher. *Arch. Biochem. Biophys.* 274(2): 532–8.

Di Matteo, V. & Esposito, E. (2003). Biochemical and therapeutic effects of antioxidants in the treatment of Alzheimer's disease, Parkinson's disease, and amyotrophic lateral sclerosis. *Curr Drug Targets CNS Neurol Disord.* 2(2): 95–107.

Diehm, C., Trampisch, H.J., Lange, S. & Schmidt, C. (1996, February). Comparison of leg compression stocking and oral horse-chestnut seed extract therapy in patients with chronic venous insufficiency. *Lancet.* 347(8997): 292–294.

Dietz, K., Jacob, S., Oelze, M., Laxa, M., Tognetti, V., de Miranda, S., Baier, M. & Finkemeier, I. (2006). The function of peroxiredoxins in plant organelle redox metabolism. *J Exp Bot.* 57(8): 1697–709.

Dimitroula, H.V., Hatzitolios, A.I. & Karvounis, H.I. (2008). The role of uric acid in stroke. *The Neurologist.* 14(4): 238–42.

Dinorah, J. (2011). Anti-inflammatory and cartilage protective effects of punicalagin, a major hydrolyzable tannin isolated from pomegranate, and a crude red raspberry extract in vitro and in vivo. *Dissertations and Master's Theses from the University of Rhode Island.* Kingston: University of Rhode Island. http://digitalcommons.uri.edu/dissertations/ AAI1508077

Dioguardi, F.S. (2008, November-December). Nutrition and skin: Collagen integrity: a dominant role for amino acids. *Clin Dermatol.* 26(6):636-40.

Dodd, S., Dean, O., Copolov, D.L., Malhi, G.S. & Berk, M. (2008). N-acetylcysteine for antioxidant therapy: pharmacology and clinical utility. *Expert Opin Biol Ther.* 8(12): 1955–62.

Doheny, K. (2011, May 3). Study: Fat May Return After Liposuction: Researchers Say Fat May Come Back 1 Year After Having the Cosmetic Procedure. http://www.webmd.com/healthy-beauty/news/20110503/study-fat-may-return-after-liposuction

Dollwet, H.H.A. & Sorenson, J.R.J. (1985). History uses of copper compounds in medicine. *Trace Elements in Medicine.* 2(2): 80 – 87.

Dorsey-Straff, N. (2010, April 30). 15 Ways to Fight, Fix and Minimize Cellulite. http://www.thatsfit.com/2010/04/30/fight-fix-and-minimize-cellulite/

Dorsey-Straff, N. (2010, March 24). The GRID: One Tool to Strengthen and Stretch. http://www.thatsfit.com/2010/03/24/the-grid-strenghten-and-stretch/

Dorsey-Straff, N. (2009, November 23). Foam Roller Exercises: Reduce Cellulite, Strengthen Your Core and More. http://www.thatsfit.com/2009/11/23/foam-roller-exercises-reduce-cellulite-core-abdominal-strength/

Doyle, C., Kushi, L.H., Byers, T. *et al.* (2006). The 2006 Nutrition, Physical Activity and Cancer Survivorship Advisory Committee. American Cancer Society. Nutrition and physical activity during and after cancer treatment: an American Cancer Society guide for informed choices. *CA Cancer J Clin.* 56:323-353.

Draelos, Z.D. (2010). Cosmeceuticals. *Body Rejuvenation.* Springer: New York.

Drake, V.J. (2010, March). Macronutrient Information Center: Manganese. http://lpi.oregonstate.edu/infocenter/minerals/manganese/

Drake, V.J. (2010, March). Macronutrient Information Center: Copper. http://lpi.oregonstate.edu/infocenter/minerals/copper/

Dresher, W.H. (2006, June). Copper and Your Skin: Facelift In A Bottle/Copper Applications in Health and Environment Area http://www.copper.org/publications/newsletters/innovations/2006/06/copper_your_skin.html

Dry Skin Brushing. (Retrieved 2012). http://www.detoxvortex.com/dryskinbrushing.html

Dry Skin Brushing. (Retrieved 2012). http://www.healingnaturallybybee.com/articles/treat7.php

Duarte, T.L. & Lunec, J. (2005). Review: When is an antioxidant not an antioxidant? A review of novel actions and reactions of vitamin C. *Free Radic. Res.* 39(7): 671–86.

Duffy, S.J. & Vita, J.A. (2003, February). Effects of phenolics on vascular endothelial function. *Curr. Opin. Lipidol.* 14(1): 21–7.

Dutta, T. & Basu, U.P. (1968). Crude extract of Centella asiatica and products derived from its glycosides as oral antifertility agents. *Indian J Exp Biol.* 6:181-2.

Duyff, R.L. (2006). *American Dietetic Association Complete Food and Nutrition Guide.* John Wiley.

Eck, J.C. & Marvel, C.S. (1943). dl-Lysine Hydrochlorides Organic Syntheses, 2:374. http://www.orgsyn.org/orgsyn/pdfs/CV2P0374.pdf

Ector, B.J., Magee, J.B., Hegwood, C.P. & Coign, M.J. (1996). Resveratrol concentration in muscadine berries, juice, pomace, purees, seeds, and wines. *American Society for Enology and Viticulture.* http://www.ajevonline.org/content/47/1/57.abstract

Elden, H.R. (1964, May 25). Hydration of connective tissue and tendon elasticity. *Biochimica et Biophysica Acta (BBA) - Specialized Section on Biophysical Subjects.* (79)3: 592–599.

Elizingre, L. (2009, October 18). How to Stop Sagging Neck Skin. http://suite101.com/article/how-to-stop-sagging-wrinkling-neck-skin-a159117

Ellagic Acid. (2008, November 1). http://www.cancer.org/Treatment/TreatmentsandSideEffects/ComplementaryandAlternativeMedicine/DietandNutrition/ellagic-acid

Ellagic Acid: Uses, Side Effects, Interactions and Warnings. (Retrieved 2012). http://www.webmd.com/vitamins-supplements/ingredientmono-1074-ELLAGIC%20ACID.aspx?activeIngredientId=1074&activeIngredientName=ELLAGIC%20ACID

Ellagic Acid Alternative Cancer Treatment Comparison. (Retrieved 2012). http://alternativecancer.us/ellagicacid.htm

Elmali, N., Baysal, O., Harma, A., Esenkaya, I. & Mizrak, B. (2007, April). Effects of resveratrol in inflammatory arthritis. *Inflammation.* 30 (1–2): 1–6.

El-Sohemy, A., Baylin, A., Kabagambe, E., Ascherio, A., Spiegelman, D. & Campos, H. (2002). Individual carotenoid concentrations in adipose tissue and plasma as biomarkers of dietary intake. *The American Journal of Clinical Nutrition.* 76(1): 172–9. http://ajcn.nutrition.org/content/76/1/172.long

Estrela, J. (2010, July 8). What Are the Dangers of Apple Cider Vinegar? http://www.livestrong.com/article/168975-what-are-the-dangers-of-apple-cider-vinegar/

Etminan, M., Takkouche, B. & Caamano-Isorna, F. (2006). The role of tomato products and lycopene in the prevention of prostate cancer: a meta-analysis of observational studies. *Cancer Epidemiol Biomarkers Prev.* 13:340-345.

Evangeliou, A. & Vlassopoulos, D. (2003). Carnitine metabolism and deficit – When supplementation is necessary? *Current Pharmaceutical Biotechnology.* 4(3): 211-219.

Faber, A.C. & Chiles, T.C. (2006, December). Resveratrol induces apoptosis in transformed follicular lymphoma OCI-LY8 cells: evidence for a novel mechanism involving inhibition of BCL6 signaling. *Int. J. Oncol.* 29(6): 1561–6. http://www.spandidos-publications.com/ijo/article.jsp?article_id=ijo_29_6_1561

Facial Exercises for a Youthful Appearance. (2012, March 24). http://www.face-wrinkles.org/facial-exercises.html

Falsaperla, M., Morgia, G., Tartarone, A., Ardito, R. & Romano, G. (2005). Support ellagic acid therapy in patients with hormone refractory prostate cancer (HRPC) on standard chemotherapy using vinorelbine and estramustine phosphate. *Eur Urol.* 47:449-454.

Farina, A., Ferranti, C. & Marra, C. (2006, March). An improved synthesis of resveratrol. *Nat. Prod. Res.* 20(3): 247–52.

Farooqi, I.S., Keogh, J.M., Kamath, S., Jones, S., Gibson, W.T., Trussell, R., Jebb, S.A., Lip, G.Y. & O'Rahilly, S. (2001, November 1). Partial leptin deficiency and human adiposity. *Nature.* 414(6859):34-5.

Farooqi, I.S. & O'Rahilly, S. (2008, October). Mutations in ligands and receptors of the leptin-melanocortin pathway that lead to obesity. *Nat Clin Pract Endocrinol Metab.* 4(10):569-77.

Farrer-Halls, G. (2005). *The Aromatherapy Bible: The Definitive Guide to Using Essential Oils.* Sterling Publishing.

Hayes, F. (Retrieved 2012). Fat on the Inside: Looking Thin is Not Enough. http://lowfatcooking.about.com/od/healthandfitness/a/bodyfat.htm

Faust, I.M., Johnson, P.R., Stern, J.R. & Hirsch, J. (1978). Diet-induced adipocyte number increase in adult rats: a new model of obesity. *AM J Physiol.* 235(3): 279–96.

Favaron, F., Lucchetta, M., Odorizzi, S., Pais da Cunha, A.T. & Sella, L. (2009). The role of grape polyphenols on trans-resveratrol activity against Botrytis Cinerea and of fungal laccase on the solubility of putative grape pr proteins. *Journal of Plant Pathology.* 91(3), 579-588. http://www.sipav.org/main/jpp/volumes/0309/030909.pdf

Ferrero, M.E., Bertelli, A.E., Fulgenzi, A., Pellegatta, F., Corsi, M.M., Bonfrate, M., Ferrara, F., De Caterina, R., Giovannini, L. & Bertelli, A. (1998, December). Activity in vitro of resveratrol on granulocyte and monocyte adhesion to endothelium. *Am. J. Clin. Nutr.* 68(6): 1208–14.

Ferrières, J. (2004, January). The French paradox: lessons for other countries. *Heart.* 90(1): 107–11. http://www.ncbi.nlm.nih.gov/pmc/articles/PMC1768013/

Finkel, T. & Holbrook, N.J. (2000). Oxidants, oxidative stress and the biology of ageing. *Nature.* 408(6809): 239–47.

Finkley, M.B., Appa, Y. & Bhandarkar, S. (2005). *Copper Peptide and Skin. Cosmeceuticals and Active Cosmetic, 2nd Edition.*, P. Eisner and H.I. Maibach (Eds.). New York: Marcel Dekker.

Fiorini, R., Ragni, L., Ambrosi, S., Littarru, G.P., Gratton, E. & Hazlett, T. (2008). Fluorescence studies of the interactions of ubiquinol-10 with liposomes. *Photochem. Photobiol.* 84(1): 209–14.

Firms Hips and Reduce the Cellulite. (Retrieved 2012). http://www.cellulitetreatmentsthatwork.com/firms-hips-and-reduce-the-cellulite/

Fish Oil and Your Skin. (2007). http://www.fishomega3fattyoil.com/fish-oil-skin.html

Fish Oil for Skin. (Retrieved 2012). http://fishoilbenefitsforhealth.com/fish-oil-for-skin/

Fish Oil Is Good for Your Skin, Your Heart, Your Brain, What Else? (2010, November 7). http://dianemae.hubpages.com/hub/Fish-Oil-Is-Good-for-your-skin-your-heart-your-brain-what-else

Fisher, G.J., Varani, J. & Voorhees, J.J. (2008, May). Looking older: Fibroblast collapse and therapeutic implications. *Arch Dermatol.* 144(5):666-672. http://archderm.jamanetwork.com/article.aspx?articleid=419693

Flagg, E.W., Coates, R.J. & Eley, J.W. (1994). Dietary glutathione intake in humans and the relationship between intake and plasma total glutathione level. *Nutr Cancer,* 21(1): 33–46.

Fluid Physiology: 2.1 Fluid Compartments. (Retrieved 2012). http://www.anaesthesiamcq.com/FluidBook/fl2_1.php

Fonseca, A. (2010, June 15). Seaweed Extract Benefits. http://www.livestrong.com/article/149603-seaweed-extract-benefits/

Foods for Healthy Skin. (Retrieved 2012). http://www.fitnessrepublic.com/nutrition/foods-for-healthy-skin.html#ixzz26fF83JKL

For Firmer, Smoother Skin, Try Collagen Supplements. (Retrieved 2012). http://www.kimecco.com/blog/firmer-smoother-skin-try-collagen-supplements

Four Arm Toning Exercises for Tightening Skin After Weight Loss. (2010, March 9). http://www.3fatchicks.com/four-arm-toning-exercises-for-tightening-skin-after-weight-loss/

France-Presse, A. (2011, September 12). 'Longevity gene' may be dead end: study. *The Raw Story.* http://www.rawstory.com/rs/2011/09/21/longevity-gene-may-be-dead-end-study/

Fraser, R.D. & MacRae, T.P. (1981). Unit cell and molecular connectivity in tendon collagen. *Int. J. Biol. Macromol.* 3(3): 193–200.

Fraser, R.D., MacRae, T.P. & Suzuki, E. (1979). Chain conformation in the collagen molecule. *J Mol Biol.* 129(3): 463–481.

Fraser, R. D., MacRae, T.P. & Miller, A. (1987). Molecular packing in type I collagen fibrils. *J Mol Biol.* 193(1): 115–125.

Fratzl, P. (2008). *Collagen: Structure and Mechanics.* New York: Springer.

Frei, B., Kim, M.C. & Ames, B.N. (1990, June). Ubiquinol-10 is an effective lipid-soluble antioxidant at physiological concentrations. *Proc. Natl. Acad. Sci. U.S.A.* 87(12): 4879–83.

Frémont, L., Belguendouz, L. & Delpal, S. (1999). Antioxidant activity of resveratrol and alcohol-free wine polyphenols related to LDL oxidation and polyunsaturated fatty acids. *Life Sci.* 64(26): 2511–21.

Frequently Asked Questions About Phytonutrients. (Retrieved 2012). http://www.webmd.com/diet/phytonutrients-faq

Frey, J. (2004, January). Collagen, ageing and nutrition. *Clin Chem Lab Med.* 42(1):9-12.

Gavura, Scott. (2011, November 24). Antioxidants and Exercise: More Harm Than Good? *Science-Based Medicine.* http://www.sciencebasedmedicine.org/index.php/antioxidants-and-exercise-more-harm-than-good/

Gehm, B.D., McAndrews, J.M., Chien, P.Y. & Jameson, J.L. (1997, December). Resveratrol, a polyphenolic compound found in grapes and wine, is an agonist for the estrogen receptor. *Proc. Natl. Acad. Sci. U.S.A.* 94(25): 14138–43. http://www.ncbi.nlm.nih.gov/pmc/articles/PMC28446/

German, J.B. (1999). Food processing and lipid oxidation. *Advances in Experimental Medicine and Biology.* 459: 23–50.

Gerster ,H. (1997). The potential role of lycopene for human health. *J Am Coll Nutr.* 16(2): 109–26.

Get Rid of Cellulite. (2008, November). Cocoa Butter for Cellulite and Stretch Marks. http://cellulite-battle.blogspot.com/2008/11/what-does-cocoa-butter-do-to-cellulite.html

Gibson, R., Perlas, L. & Hotz, C. (2006). Improving the bioavailability of nutrients in plant foods at the household level. *Proc Nutr Soc.* 65(2): 160–8.

Gibson, W.T., Farooqi, I.S., Moreau, M., DePaoli, A.M., Lawrence, E., O'Rahilly, S. & Trussell, R.A. (2004, October). Congenital leptin deficiency due to homozygosity for the Delta133G mutation: report of another case and evaluation of response to four years of leptin therapy. *J Clin Endocrinol Metab.* 89(10):4821-6.

Giovannucci, E., Ascherio, A., Rimm, E.B., Stampfer, M.J., Colditz, G.A. & Willett, W.C. (1995). Intake of carotenoids and retinol in relation to risk of prostate cancer. *J. Natl. Cancer Inst.* 87(23): 1767–76.

Giovannucci, E., Willett, W.C., Stampfer, M.J., Liu, Y. & Rimm, E.B. (2002). A prospective study of tomato products, lycopene, and prostate cancer risk. *J. Natl Cancer Inst.* 94(5): 391–39.

Giovannucci, E. (2005, August). Tomato products, lycopene, and prostate cancer: a review of the epidemiological literature. *J Nutr.* 135(8):2030S-1S.

Goldberg, D.M., Yan, J. & Soleas, G.J. (2003, February). Absorption of three wine-related polyphenols in three different matrices by healthy subjects. *Clin. Biochem.* 36(1): 79–87.

Goldman, M.P. (Retrieved 2012). Collagen Injections – Benefits, Cost & Side Effects. http://www.yourplasticsurgeryguide.com/injectables-and-fillers/collagen.htm

Goode, J. (Retrieved 2012). Discover the Connection Between Essential Oils and Wrinkles. http://www.sourceofenlightenment.com/Aromatherapy.html

Goodman, M., Bostick, R.M., Ward, K.C. *et al.* (2006). Lycopene intake and prostate cancer risk: effect modification by plasma antioxidants and the XRCC1 genotype. *Nutrition & Cancer.* 55:13-20.

Goodrow, E.F., Wilson, T.A. & Houde, S.C. (2006). Consumption of one egg per day increases serum lutein and zeaxanthin concentrations in older adults without altering serum lipid and lipoprotein cholesterol concentrations. *J. Nutr.* 136 (10): 2519–24.

Gorouhi, F. & Maibach, H.I. (2009). Role of topical peptides in preventing and treating aged skin. *Int. J. Cosm. Sci.* 31:327-345.

Gotu Kola. (Retrieved 2012). http://www.webmd.com/vitamins-supplements/ingredientmono-753-GOTU%20KOLA.aspx?activeIngredientId =753&activeIngredientName=GOTU%20KOLA

Grace, M., Fischer, M.D., Josep, G. & Llaurado, M.D. (1966, October). Collagen and elastin content in canine arteries selected from functionally different vascular beds. *Circulation Research.* 19(2): 394–399.

Graham, E. (2009, September 21). Kinetin - Mother Nature's Wonder-Extract. http://ezinearticles.com/?Kinetin---Mother-Natures-Wonder-Extract&id= 2867242

Graham, J.S., Stevenson, R.S., Mitcheltree, L.W., Hamilton, A., Deckert, R.R., Lee, R.B & Schiavetta, A.M. (2009). U.S. Army Medical Research Institute of Chemical Defense. Medical management of cutaneous sulfur mustard injuries. *Toxicology.* 263, 47-58.

Grape Seed Extract: Dosage, Precautions and Interactions. (Retrieved 2012). http://en.wikipedia.org/wiki/Grape_seed_extract#Dosage.2C_precautions_and_ interactions

Grape Seed Extract and the Prevention of Chronic Degenerative Disease. (Retrieved 2012). http://www.preventive-health-guide.com/grape-seed-extract.html

Grape Seed Extract Benefits. (Retrieved 2012). http://www.buzzle.com/articles/ grape-seed-extract-benefits.html

Grape Seed. (2011). http://www.umm.edu/altmed/articles/grape-seed-000254.htm

Green, D.E. & Tzagoloff, A. (1966, September). The mitochondrial electron transfer chain. *Arch. Biochem. Biophys.* 116(1): 293–304.

Green, G.A. (2008). Review: antioxidant supplements do not reduce all-cause mortality in primary or secondary prevention. *Evid Based Med.* 13(6): 177.

Griffith, R.S., Norins, A.L. & Kagan, C. (1978). A multicentered study of lysine therapy in Herpes simplex infection. *Dermatologica.* 156(5): 257–267.

Grossman, A.R., Lohr, M. & Im, C.S. (2004). Chlamydomonas reinhardtii in the landscape of pigments. *Annu. Rev. Genet.* 38(1): 119–73.

Grossman, R. (2005). The role of dimethylaminoethanol in cosmetic dermatology. *Am J Clin Dermatol*, 6(1):39-47. http://www.ncbi.nlm.nih.gov/pubmed/15675889

Group, E.F. (2010, March 9). 11 Foods High in Calcium. http://www.globalhealingcenter.com/natural-health/foods-high-in-calcium/

Gruber, J., Tang, S.Y. & Halliwell, B. (2007, April). Evidence for a trade-off between survival and fitness caused by resveratrol treatment of Caenorhabditis elegans. *Ann. N. Y. Acad. Sci.* 1100: 530–42.

Gu, X., Creasy, L., Kester, A. & Zeece, M. (1999, August). Capillary electrophoretic determination of resveratrol in wines. *J. Agric. Food Chem.* 47(8): 3223–7.

Gul, N.Y., Topal, A., Cangul, I.T. & Yanik, K. (2008). The effects of topical tripeptide copper complex and helium-neon laser on wound healing in rabbits. *Vet Dermatol.* 19(1):7-14.

Guo, J.S., Cheng, C.L. & Koo, M.W. (2004). Inhibitory effects of Centella asiatica water extract and asiaticoside on inducible nitric oxide synthase during gastric ulcer healing in rats. *Planta Med.* 70:1150-4.

Guyton, A.C. (1986). *Textbook of Medical Physiology.* Philadelphia: W.B. Saunders.

Guyton, A.C. (1991). *Textbook of Medical Physiology* (8th ed.). Philadelphia: W.B. Saunders.

Haider, U.G., Roos, T.U., Kontaridis, M.I., Neel, B.G., Sorescu, D., Griendling, K.K., Vollmar, A.M. & Dirsch, V.M. (2005, July). Resveratrol inhibits angiotensin II- and epidermal growth factor-mediated Akt activation: role of Gab1 and Shp2. *Mol. Pharmacol.* 68(1): 41–8.

Hail, N., Cortes, M., Drake, E.N. & Spallholz, J.E. (2008). Cancer chemoprevention: a radical perspective. *Free Radic. Biol. Med.* 45(2): 97–110.

Hall, G.P. (Retrieved 2012). For Vitamins and Sagging Skin – You Could Try Grape Seed Oil and Co-Enzyme Q10. http://ezinearticles.com/?For-Vitamins-and-Sagging-Skin---You-Could-Try-Grape-Seed-Oil-and-Coenzyme-Q10&id=4553628

Halliwell, B. (2008). Are polyphenols antioxidants or pro-oxidants? What do we learn from cell culture and in vivo studies? *Archives of Biochemistry and Biophysics.* 476(2): 107–112.

Hampton, J. (2009, October 27). Facial Skin Tightening Exercises. http://www.livestrong.com/article/22105-facial-skin-tightening-exercises/

Haseen, F., Cantwell, M.M., O'Sullivan, J.M. & Murray, L.J. (2009). Is there a benefit from lycopene supplementation in men with prostate cancer? A systematic review. *Prostate Cancer Prostatic Dis.* 12(4):325-32.

Hausen, B.M. (1993). Centella asiatica (Indian pennywort), an effective therapeutic but a weak sensitizer. *Contact Dermatitis.* 29:175-9.

Haycock, D.A. (2011, July 18). Green Tea Helps Your Skin Stay Younger. http://www.fyiliving.com/health/green-tea-helps-your-skin-stay-younger/

Hays, N.P., Kim, H., Wells, A.M., Kajkenova, O. & Evans, W.J. (2009, June). Effects of whey and fortified collagen hydrolysate protein supplements on nitrogen balance and body composition in older women. *J Am Diet Assoc.* 109(6):1082-7.

Healing Daily: Vitamin C. (2002). http://www.healingdaily.com/detoxification-diet/vitamin-c.htm

Health Benefits of Rebounding. (Retrieved 2012). http://www.squidoo.com/health-benefits-of-rebounding

Hellesvig-Gaskell, K. (Retrieved 2012). Salicylic Acid Dangers. http://www.ehow.com/facts_5285090_salicylic-acid-dangers.html

Herbal remedies using pennywort (Centella asiatica). (Retrieved 2012). http://www.ageless.co.za/pennywort.htm

Herbal Therapeutics: Natural Skin Supplements. (Retrieved 2012). http://www.herbal-therapeutics.com/skin-supplements.html

Hercberg, S., Galan, P., Preziosi, P., Bertrais, S., Mennen, L., Malvy, D., Roussel, A.M., Favier, A. & Briancon, S. (2004). The SU.VI.MAX Study: a randomized, placebo-controlled trial of the health effects of antioxidant vitamins and minerals. *Arch Intern Med.* 164(21): 2335–42.

Herrera, E. & Barbas, C. (2001). Vitamin E: Action, metabolism and perspectives. *Journal of Physiology and Biochemistry.* 57(2): 43–56.

Higdon, J., Drake, V.J. & Steward, W.P. (2008, May). Resveratrol. *Micronutrient Information Center.* Linus Pauling Institute.

Himms-Hagen, J. (1990). Brown adipose tissue thermogenesis: Interdisciplinary studies. *FASEB Journal: Official Publication of the Federation of American Societies for Experimental Biology.* 4(11): 2890–8.

Ho, Y.S., Magnenat, J.L., Gargano, M. & Cao, J. (1998). The nature of antioxidant defense mechanisms: a lesson from transgenic studies. *Environ. Health Perspect.* 106 (Suppl 5): 1219–28. http://www.ncbi.nlm.nih.gov/pmc/articles/PMC1533365/

Holmes, D. F., Gilpin, C. J., Baldock, C., Ziese, U., Koster, A. J. & Kadler, K. E. (2001). Corneal collagen fibril structure in three dimensions: Structural insights into fibril assembly, mechanical properties, and tissue organization. *PNAS.* 98(13): 7307–7312.

Holmes, D.F. & Kadler, K.E. (2006). The 10+4 microfibril structure of thin cartilage fibrils. *PNAS.* 103(46): 17249–17254.

Home Remedy Central. (Retrieved 2012). Cellulite. http://www.homeremedycentral.com/en/natural-cures/home-remedy/cellulite.html

Hornig, D., Vuilleumier, J. & Hartmann, D. (1980). Absorption of large, single, oral intakes of ascorbic acid. *Int J Vitam Nutr Res.* 50(3): 309–14.

Horse Chestnut: Benefits and Side Effects. (Retrieved 2012). http://vitamins.ultimatefatburner.com/horse-chestnut.html

Hosoe, K., Kitano, M., Kishida, H., Kubo, H., Fujii, K. & Kitahara, M. (2007, February). Study on safety and bioavailability of ubiquinol (Kaneka QH) after single and 4-week multiple oral administration to healthy volunteers. *Regul. Toxicol. Pharmacol.* 47(1): 19–28.

Houck, J.C., Sharma, V.K., Patel, Y.M. & Gladner, J.A. (1968). Induction of collagenolytic and proteolytic activities by anti-inflammatory drugs in the skin and fibroblasts. *Biochemical Pharmacology.* 17(10): 2081–2090.

How Methylxanthines Work on Cellulites. (2012, July 6). http://topcellulitetreatmentguide.com/how-methylxanthines-work-on-cellulites/

How to Choose Collagen Supplements: Navigating the World of Collagen Supplements, from Gucosamine and Chondroitin to Liquid Vitamins. (Retrieved 2012). http://www.howtodothings.com/health-and-fitness/a4460-how-to-choose-collagen-supplements.html

How to Clear and Tighten Skin With Rebound Exercise. (Retrieved 2012). http://www.ehow.com/how_2065897_clear-tighten-skin-rebound-exercise.html

How to Easily Get Rid of Cellulite. (Retrieved 2012). http://www.ehow.com/how_5823444_easily-rid-cellulite.html

How To Increase Collagen In the Body. (Retrieved 2012). http://collagenman.hubpages.com/hub/How-To-Increase-Collagen-In-the-Body

How to Repair Connective Tissue. (Retrieved 2012). http://www.tryfosstherapies.com.au/Tryfoss_Therapies/Repairing_Connective_Tissue.html

How to Tighten Skin With Dry Brushing. (Retrieved 2012). http://www.ehow.com/how_4454623_tighten-skin-dry-brushing.html

Hulmes, D.J. & Miller, A. (1979). Quasi-hexagonal molecular packing in collagen fibrils. *Nature.* 282(5741): 878–880.

Hulmes, D.J. (1992). The collagen superfamily—diverse structures and assemblies. *Essays Biochem.* 27: 49–67.

Hulmes, D.J. (2002). Building collagen molecules, fibrils, and suprafibrillar structures. *J Struct Biol.* 137(1–2): 2–10.

Hunt, J. (2003). Bioavailability of iron, zinc, and other trace minerals from vegetarian diets. *Am J Clin Nutr.* 78(3 Suppl): 633S–639S. http://ajcn.nutrition.org/content/78/3/633S.full

Hurrell, R. (2003). Influence of vegetable protein sources on trace element and mineral bioavailability. *J Nutr.* 133(9): 2973S–7S. http://jn.nutrition.org/content/133/9/2973S.full

Hurst, W.J., Glinski, J.A., Miller, K.B., Apgar, J., Davey, M.H. & Stuart, D.A. (2008, September). Survey of the trans-resveratrol and trans-piceid content of cocoa-containing and chocolate products. *J. Agric. Food Chem.* 56(18): 8374–8.

Imlay, J.A. (2003). Pathways Ofoxidativedamage. *Annual Review of Microbiology.* 57:395–418.

Incandela, L., Belcaro, G., Cesarone, M.R. *et al.* (2001). Treatment of diabetic microangiopathy and edema with total triterpenic fraction of Centella asiatica: a prospective, placebo-controlled randomized study. *Angiology.* 52 Suppl 2:S27-31.

Incandela, L., Belcaro, G., De Sanctis, M.T. *et al.* (2001). Total triterpenic fraction of Centella asiatica in the treatment of venous hypertension: a clinical, prospective, randomized trial using a combined microcirculatory model. *Angiology.* 52 Suppl 2:S61-7.

Incandela, L., Belcaro, G., Nicolaides, A.N. *et al.* (2001). Modification of the echogenicity of femoral plaques after treatment with total triterpenic fraction of Centella asiatica: a prospective, randomized, placebo-controlled trial. *Angiology.* 52 Suppl 2:S69-73.

Incandela, L., Cesarone, M.R., Cacchio, M. *et al.* (2001). Total triterpenic fraction of Centella asiatica in chronic venous insufficiency and in high-perfusion microangiopathy. *Angiology.* 52 Suppl 2:S9-13.

Institute of Medicine of the National Academies. (2002, September 5). Dietary Reference Intakes for Macronutrients. http://www.iom.edu/Reports/2002/Dietary-Reference-Intakes-for-Energy-Carbohydrate-Fiber-Fat-Fatty-Acids-Cholesterol-Protein-and-Amino-Acids.aspx

Irving, D.C., Brock, D., Weltman, J., Swift, D., Barrett, E., Gaesser, G. & Weltman, A. (2008). Effect of exercise training intensity on abdominal visceral fat and body composition. *Medicine and Science in Sports and Exercise.* 40(11): 1863–1872.

Ishikawa, A., Kawarazaki, H., Ando, K., Fujita, M., Fujita, T. & Homma, Y. (2011, February). Renal preservation effect of ubiquinol, the reduced form of coenzyme Q10. *Clin. Exp. Nephrol.* 15(1): 30–3.

Jacob, R.A. (1996). Three eras of vitamin C discovery. *Sub-Cellular Biochemistry.* 25: 1–16.

Jacques, E. (2011, May 18). What Are the Dangers of Beta Carotene? http://www.livestrong.com/article/444960-what-are-the-dangers-of-beta-carotene/

Jakeman, P. & Maxwell, S. (1993). Effect of antioxidant vitamin supplementation on muscle function after eccentric exercise. *Eur J Appl Physiol Occup Physiol.* 67(5): 426–30.

Jang, M., Cai, L., Udeani, G.O., Slowing, K.V., Thomas, C.F., Beecher, C.W., Fong, H.H., Farnsworth, N.R., Kinghorn, A.D., Mehta, R.G., Moon, R.C. & Pezzuto, J.M. (1997, January). Cancer chemopreventive activity of resveratrol, a natural product derived from grapes. *Science.* 275(5297): 218–20.

Jatoi, A., Burch, P., Hillman, D. *et al.* (2007). A tomato-based, lycopene-containing intervention for androgen-independent prostate cancer: results of a Phase II study from the North Central Cancer Treatment Group. *Urology.* 69:289-294.

Jean-Gilles, D. (2011). Anti-inflammatory and cartilage protective effects of punicalagin, a major hydrolysable tannin isolated from pomegranate, and a crude red raspberry extract in vitro and in vivo. *Dissertations and Master's Theses From the University of Rhode Island.* Kingston: University of Rhode Island.

Jepsen, P. (Retrieved 2012). Cellulite Treatment Cream Using Caffeine. http://pierjepsen.hubpages.com/hub/Cellulite-Treatment-Cream-Using-Caffeine

Jesior, J.C., Miller, A. & Berthet-Colominas, C. (1980). Crystalline three-dimensional packing is general characteristic of type I collagen fibrils. *FEBS Lett.* 113(2): 238–240.

Jha, P., Flather, M., Lonn, E., Farkouh, M. & Yusuf, S. (1995). The antioxidant vitamins and cardiovascular disease: A critical review of epidemiologic and clinical trial data. *Annals of Internal Medicine.* 123(11): 860–872.

JKL Company. The JKL Vitamin Guide. (Retrieved 2012). http://www.jklcompany.com/13301.html

Jo, J.Y., Gonzalez de Mejia, E. & Lila, M.A. (2006, March). Catalytic inhibition of human DNA topoisomerase II by interactions of grape cell culture polyphenols. *J. Agric. Food Chem.* 54(6): 2083–7.

Jogging Is Bad For the Skin – What About Rebounding? (2010, May 8). http://rebounding.tv/jogging-is-bad-for-the-skin-what-about-rebounding/

Hansen, J.T. & Koeppen, B.M. (2002). *Netter's Atlas of Human Physiology.* Teterboro, N.J: Icon Learning Systems.

Johnson, F. & Giulivi, C. (2005). Superoxide dismutases and their impact upon human health. *Mol Aspects Med.* 26(4–5): 340–52.

Johnson, R.J., Andrews, P., Benner, S.A. & Oliver, W. (2010). Theodore E. Woodward award. The evolution of obesity: Insights from the mid-Miocene. *Transactions of the American Clinical and Climatological Association.* 121: 295–305, discussion 305–8. http://www.ncbi.nlm.nih.gov/pmc/articles/PMC2917125/

Jones, A. (Retrieved 2012). What Vitamins Are Needed for Skin Elasticity? http://www.ehow.com/about_5484929_vitamins-needed-skin-elasticity.html#ixzz26fFUXlks

Jones, C. (2010, April 27). Alpha & Beta Hydroxy Acids. http://www.livestrong.com/article/112874-alpha-beta-hydroxy-acids/

Jönsson, T.J. & Lowther, W.T. (2007). The peroxiredoxin repair proteins. *Subcellular Biochemistry.* 44: 115–41. http://www.ncbi.nlm.nih.gov/pmc/articles/PMC2391273/

Jordan-Reilly, M. (2011, June 14). Minerals Needed to Keep Skin Firm. http://www.livestrong.com/article/267447-minerals-needed-to-keep-skin-firm/

Jorge, O.A. & Jorge, A.D. (2005). Hepatotoxicity associated with the ingestion of Centella asiatica. *Rev Esp Enferm Dig,* 97:115-24.

Kaeberlein, M., McDonagh, T., Heltweg, B., Hixon, J., Westman, E.A., Caldwell, S.D., Napper, A., Curtis, R., DiStefano, P.S., Fields, S., Bedalov, A. & Kennedy, B.K. (2005, April). Substrate-specific activation of sirtuins by resveratrol. *J. Biol. Chem.* 280(17): 17038–45.

Khan, M.A., Tania, M., Zhang, D. & Chen, H. (2010). Antioxidant enzymes and cancer. *Chin J Cancer Res.* 22(2): 87–92. http://www.springerlink.com/content/4h2277984v0t180k/?MUD=MP

Khan, N., Afaq, F. & Mukhtar, H. (2008). Cancer chemoprevention through dietary antioxidants: progress and promise. *Antioxid. Redox Signal.* 10(3): 475–510.

Khaw, K. & Woodhouse, P. (1995). Interrelation of vitamin C, infection, haemostatic factors, and cardiovascular disease. *BMJ.* 310 (6994): 1559–63. http://www.bmj.com/content/310/6994/1559?view=long &pmid=7787643

Kielty, C.M., Sherratt M.J. & Shuttleworth C.A. (2002, July). Elastic fibres. *J. Cell. Sci.* 115(Pt 14): 2817–28.

Kinetin: A Wonder Ingredient In Skin Care? (2009, August 11). http://blog.pharmacymix.com/kinetin-a-wonder-ingredient-in-skin-care

King, D. (2011, October 11). Connective Tissue Study Guide. Southern Illinois University School of Medicine. http://www.siumed.edu/~dking2/intro/ct.htm#4.4

Kirsh, V.A., Mayne, S.T., Peters, U. *et al.* (2006). A prospective study of lycopene and tomato product intake and risk of prostate cancer. *Cancer Epidemiology, Biomarkers & Prevention.* 15:92-98.

Knight, J.A. (1998). Free radicals: Their history and current status in aging and disease. *Annals of Clinical and Laboratory Science.* 28(6): 331–46.

Kondo, T., Kishi, M., Fushimi, T. & Kaga, T. (2009, July 8). Acetic acid upregulates the expression of genes for fatty acid oxidation enzymes in liver to suppress body fat accumulation. *J. Agric. Food Chem.* 57(13): 5982-6.

Kopp, P. (1998, June). Resveratrol, a phytoestrogen found in red wine. A possible explanation for the conundrum of the 'French paradox'? *Eur. J. Endocrinol.* 138(6): 619–2.

Kresty, L.A., Morse, M.A., Morgan, C. *et al.* (2001). Chemoprevention of esophageal tumorigenesis by dietary administration of lyophilized black raspberries. *Cancer Res.* 61:6112-6119.

Kubo, H., Fujiib, K., Kawabea, T., Matsumotoa, S., Kishidaa, H. & Hosoea, K. (2008, May). Food Content of ubiquinol-10 and ubiquinone-10 in the Japanese diet. *Journal of Food Composition and Analysis.* 21(3): 199–210.

Kumar, P., Padi, S.S., Naidu, P.S. & Kumar, A. (2006, September). Effect of resveratrol on 3-nitropropionic acid-induced biochemical and behavioural changes: possible neuroprotective mechanisms. *Behav Pharmacol.* 17(5–6): 485–92.

Kuo, L. *et al.* (2008). Associations between periodontal diseases and systemic diseases: a review of the inter-relationships and interactions with diabetes, respiratory diseases, cardiovascular diseases, and osteoporosis. *Public Health*, 122, 417-433

Kushi, L.H., Byers, T., Doyle, C. *et al.* (2006). American Cancer Society Guidelines on Nutrition and Physical Activity for cancer prevention: reducing the risk of cancer with healthy food choices and physical activity. *CA Cancer J Clin.* 56:254-281.

Labrecque, L., Lamy, S., Chapus, A. *et al.* (2005). Combined inhibition of PDGF and VEGF receptors by ellagic acid, a dietary-derived phenolic compound. *Carcinogenesis.* 26:821-826.

Lai, P.B., Zhang, L. & Yang, L.Y. (2011, October 20). Quercetin ameliorates diabetic nephropathy by reducing the expressions of transforming growth factor-β1 and connective tissue growth factor in streptozotocin-induced diabetic rats. *Ren Fail.* 34(1):83-7. http://www.ncbi.nlm.nih.gov/pubmed/22011322

Lamb, J. (2007). The connectivity map: A new tool for biomedical research. *Nat. Rev. Cancer.* 7(1):54-60.

Lammers, S.R., Kao, P.H., Qi, H.J., Hunter, K., Lanning, C., Albietz, J., Hofmeister, S., Mecham, R., Stenmark, K.R. & Shandas, R. (2008, July). Changes in the structure-function relationship of elastin and its impact on the proximal pulmonary arterial mechanics of hypertensive calves. *Am J Physiol Heart Circ Physiol.* 295(4): H1451-9.

Lamont, K.T., Somers, S., Lacerda, L., Opie, L.H. & Lecour, S. (2011, May). Is red wine a SAFE sip away from cardioprotection? Mechanisms involved in resveratrol- and melatonin-induced cardioprotection. *J. Pineal Res.* 50(4): 374–80.

Lampert, L. (2011, July 27). Dangerous Side Effects of Resveratrol. http://www.livestrong.com/article/502666-dangerous-side-effects-of-resveratrol/

Langella, F. (Retrieved 2012). How to Firm Up Sagging Neck Skin? And Other FAQs. http://www.articledashboard.com/Article/How-to-Firm-Up-Sagging-Neck-Skin-and-Other-FAQs/958469

Langsjoen, P.H. et al. (2010, May 27-30). Supplemental Ubiquinol in congestive heart failure - 3 year experience. *Sixth Conference of the International Coenzyme Q10 Association*. Brussels, Belgium.

Langsjoen, P.H. & Langsjoen, A.M. (2008). Supplemental ubiquinol in patients with advanced congestive heart failure. *BioFactors*. 32(1-4): 119–28.

Larrosa, M., Tomás-Barberán, F.A. & Espín, J.C. (2006). The dietary hydrolysable tannin punicalagin releases ellagic acid that induces apoptosis in human colon adenocarcinoma Caco-2 cells by using the mitochondrial pathway. *The Journal of Nutritional Biochemistry*. 17(9): 611–625.

Laskin, J.D. (1999, October). *Conference on the Advances in the Biology and Treatment of Skin: Final Proceedings*. University of Medicine and Dentistry of New Jersey. Piscataway, N.J.

Lawenda, B.D., Kelly, K.M., Ladas, E.J., Sagar, S.M., Vickers, A. & Blumberg, J.B. (2008). Should supplemental antioxidant administration be avoided during chemotherapy and radiation therapy? *J Natl Cancer Inst*. 100: 773-783.

LeBlanc, M.R. (2005, December 13). *Cultivar, Juice Extraction, Ultra Violet Irradiation and Storage Influence the Stilbene Content of Muscadine Grapes (Vitis Rotundifolia Michx.)*. Louisiana State University: Baton Rouge.

Ledford, H. (2011). Longevity genes challenged. *Nature*.

Lee, I.M., Cook, N.R. & Gaziano, J.M. (2005). Vitamin E in the primary prevention of cardiovascular disease and cancer: the Women's Health Study: a randomized controlled trial. *JAMA* 294 (1): 56–65.

Lee, T., Kim, S., Yu, S., Kim, S., Park, D., Moon, H., Dho, S., Kwon, K., Kwon, H., Han, Y., Jeong, S., Kang, S., Shin, H., Lee, K., Rhee, S. & Yu, D. (2003). Peroxiredoxin II is essential for sustaining life span of erythrocytes in mice. *Blood*. 101(12): 5033–8. http://bloodjournal.hematologylibrary.org/content/101/12/5033.full

Leeuwenburgh, C., Fiebig, R., Chandwaney, R. & Ji, L. (1994). Aging and exercise training in skeletal muscle: responses of glutathione and antioxidant enzyme systems. *Am J Physiol*. 267 (2 Pt 2): R439–45. http://ajpregu.physiology.org/content/267/2/R439.full.pdf+html

Leeuwenburgh, C. & Heinecke, J. (2001). Oxidative stress and antioxidants in exercise. *Curr Med Chem*. 8 (7): 829–38.

Lemerond, T. (2011). How Silica Strengthens Bones, Firms Skin and Enhances Beauty! http://www.terrytalksnutrition.com/weekly-articles/2010/07-30/how-silica-strengthens-bones-firms-skin-and-enhances-beauty/

Lenaz, G., Fato R., Di Bernardo S. et al. (1999). Localization and mobility of coenzyme Q in lipid bilayers and membranes. *BioFactors*. 9(2-4): 87–93.

Leone, S., Cornetta, T., Basso, E. & Cozzi, R. (2010, September). Resveratrol induces DNA double-strand breaks through human topoisomerase II interaction. *Cancer Lett*. 295(2): 167–72.

Leong, K. (Retrieved 2012). Copper Peptides as Treatment for Aging Facial Skin: Do They Work? http://voices.yahoo.com/copper-peptides-as-treatment-aging-facial-skin-1859864.html?cat=69

Levi, F., Pasche, C., Lucchini, F., Ghidoni, R., Ferraroni, M. & La Vecchia, C. (2005, April). Resveratrol and breast cancer risk. *Eur. J. Cancer Prev.* 14(2): 139–42.

Levy, J., Sharoni, Y., Danilenko, M., Miinster, A., Bosin, E., Giat, Y. & Feldman, B. (1995). Lycopene is a more potent inhibitor of human cancer cell proliferation than either alpha-carotene or beta-carotene. *Nutr Cancer.* 24 (3): 257–266.

Leyden, J., Stephens, T., Finkey, M.B., Appa, Y. & Barkovic, S. (2002, February). Skin Care Benefits of Copper Peptide Containing Facial Cream. *Amer Academy Dermat Meeting.* 68-69.

Lin, K.H., Hsiao, G., Shih, C.M., Chou, D.S. & Sheu, J.R. (2009). Mechanisms of resveratrol-induced platelet apoptosis. *Cardiovascular research.* 83(3): 575–85.

Linster, C.L. & Van Schaftingen, E. (2007). Vitamin C. *FEBS Journal.* 274(1): 1–22.

Littel, R.J., Bos, M. & Knoop, G.J. (1990). Dissociation constants of some alkanolamines at 293, 303, 318, and 333 K. *J. Chem. Eng. Data.* 35: 276–277.

Litwack, G. (2008). *Human Biochemistry and Disease.* Academic Press.

Liu, X., Zhao, Y., Gao, J. *et al.* (2004, February). Elastic fiber homeostasis requires lysyl oxidase-like 1 protein. *Nat. Genet.* 36(2): 178–82.

Lombard, D.B., Pletcher, S.D., Cantó, C. & Auwerx, J. (2011, September). Ageing: longevity hits a roadblock. *Nature.* 477(7365): 410–1.

Lopes, L.B., VanDeWall, H., Li, H.T., Venugopal, V., Li, H.K., Naydin, S., Hosmer, J., Levendusky, M., Zheng, H., Bentley, M.V., Levin, R. & Hass, M.A. (2010, March). Topical delivery of lycopene using microemulsions: enhanced skin penetration and tissue antioxidant activity. *J Pharm Sci.* 99(3):1346-57. http://www.ncbi.nlm.nih.gov/pubmed/19798758

Lotito, S.B. & Frei, B. (2006). Consumption of flavonoid-rich foods and increased plasma antioxidant capacity in humans: cause, consequence, or epiphenomenon? *Free Radic. Biol. Med.* 41(12): 1727–46.

Lycopene. (Retrieved 2012). http://www.cancer.org/Treatment/Treatmentsand SideEffects/ComplementaryandAlternativeMedicine/DietandNutrition/lycopene

Lycopene Information. (Retrieved 2012). http://www.drugs.com/npc/lycopene.html

Lynch, W. Copper & Skin Care. (2011, June 14). http://www.livestrong.com/article/260126-copper-skin-care/#ixzz267DoNytg

Lyons, M.M., Yu, C., Toma, R.B., Cho, S.Y., Reiboldt, W., Lee, J. & van Breemen, R.B. (2003, September). Resveratrol in raw and baked blueberries and bilberries. *J. Agric. Food Chem.* 51(20): 5867–70.

Lysine. (Retrieved 2012). http://www.herbs2000.com/amino_acids/lysine.htm

M.C. Biotech, Inc. (2011, February 10). Material Safety Data Sheet: Copper Peptide. http://www.mcbiotec.com/file/msds%20copper%20peptide.pdf

Macmillan-Crow, L.A. & Cruthirds, D.L. (2001, April). Invited review: manganese superoxide dismutase in disease. *Free Radic. Res.* 34(4): 325–36.

Madison, K.C. (2003). Barrier function of the skin: *la raison d'être* of the epidermis. *J Invest Dermatol.* 121(2):231-41.

Maeda, H., Hosokawa, M., Sashima, T., Funayama, K. & Miyashita, K. (2005, July). Fucoxanthin from edible seaweed, *Unidaria pinnatifida*, shows antiobesity effect through UCP1 expression in white adipose tissues. *Biochemical and Biophysical Research Communications.* 332(2): 392-397.

Maiani, G., Periago Castón, M.J. & Catasta, G. (2008). Carotenoids: Actual knowledge on food sources, intakes, stability and bioavailability and their protective role in humans. *Mol Nutr Food Res.* 53: S194–218.

Mallol, J., Belda, M.A. & Costa, D., *et al.* (1991). Prophylaxis of striae gravidarum with a topical formulation. A double blind trial. *Int J Cosmet Sci.* 3:51-7.

Mämmelä, P., Savolainen, H., Lindroos, L., Kangas, J. & Vartiainen, T. (2000). Analysis of oak tannins by liquid chromatography-electrospray ionisation mass spectrometry. *Journal of Chromatography A.* 891(1): 75–83.

Maquart, F.X., Bellon, G., Pasco, S. & Monboisse, J.C. (2005, March-April). Matrikines in the regulation of extracellular matrix degradation. *Biochimie.* 87(3-4):353-60

Maquart, F.X., Chastang, F., Simeon, A. *et al.* (1999). Triterpenes from Centella asiatica stimulate extracellular matrix accumulation in rat experimental wounds. *Eur J Dermatol.* 9:289-96.

Maquart, F.X., Pickart, L., Laurent, M., Gillery, P., Monboisse, J.C. & Borel, J.P. (1988). Stimulation of collagen synthesis in fibroblast cultures by the tripeptide-copper complex glycyl-L-histidyl-L-lysine-Cu2+. *FEBS Lett.* 10; 238(2):343-6.

Marambaud, P., Zhao, H. & Davies, P. (2005, November). Resveratrol promotes clearance of Alzheimer's disease amyloid-beta peptides. *J. Biol. Chem.* 280(45): 37377–82.

Marieb, E. & Hoehn, K. (2008). *Anatomy and Physiology, 3rd Edition.* Benjamin Cummings.

Marquart, F.X., Pickart, L., Laurent, M., Gillery, P., Monboisse, J.C. & Borel, J.P. (1988). Stimulation of collagen syusnthesis in fibroblast cultures by the tripeptide-copper complex glycyl-L-histidyl-L-Cu2+, *FEBS Lett.* 232(2): 343-346.

Mattill, H.A. (1947). Antioxidants. *Annual Review of Biochemistry.* 16: 177–92.

Mattivi, F. (1993, June). Solid phase extraction of trans-resveratrol from wines for HPLC analysis. *Z Lebensm Unters Forsch.* 196(6): 522–5.

Mattivi, F., Reniero, F. & Korhammer, S. (1995). Isolation, characterization, and evolution in red wine vinification of resveratrol monomers. *J Agric Food Chem.* 43(7): 1820–3.

Mature Skin. (Retrieved 2012). http://us.eminenceorganics.com/Firm-Skin-Vitamins_p_389.html

May, L. (July 19, 2010). Grape Seed Extract Offers Many Benefits. http://www.naturalnews.com/029223_grape_seed_extract_health.html

Mayo Clinic. (2011, April 16). Belly fat in women: How to keep it off. http://www.mayoclinic.com/health/belly-fat/WO00128

Mayo Clinic. (2010, October 12). Wrinkle Creams: Your Guide to Younger Looking Skin. http://www.mayoclinic.com/health/wrinkle-creams/SN00010

Mayo Clinic. (Retrieved 2012). Cellulite. http://www.mayoclinic.com/health/cellulite/DS00891

Mayo Clinic. (Retrieved 2012). DHEA. http://www.mayoclinic.com/health/dhea/NS_patient-dhea/DSECTION=evidence

Mayo Clinic. (Retrieved 2012). Lycopene. http://www.mayoclinic.com/health/lycopene/NS_patient-lycopene

Mayo Clinic. (Retrieved 2012). Nutrition and Health Eating: Do Detox Diets Offer Any Health Benefits? http://www.mayoclinic.com/health/detox-diets/AN01334

Mazurek, T., Zhang, L., Zalewski, A. *et al.* (2003, November). Human epicardial adipose tissue is a source of inflammatory mediators. *Circulation.* 108(20): 2460–6.

McAllister, C. (2011, July 5). Foods that Build Collagen & Elastin After Age 50. http://www.livestrong.com/article/485132-foods-that-build-collagen-elastin-after-age-50/#ixzz26aRyMuDT

McCormack, M.C., Nowak, K.C. & Koch, R.J. (2001). The effect of copper tripeptide and tretinoin on growth factor production in a serium-free fibroblast model. *Arch. Facial Plast. Surg.* 3: 28 – 32.

McFee, R.B., Caraccio, T.R., McGuigan, M.A., Reynolds, S.A. & Bellanger, P. (2004). Dying to be thin: A dinitrophenol related fatality. *Veterinary and human toxicology.* 46(5): 251–4.

McGee, F. (Retrieved 2012). Natural Ways to Tighten Up Skin. http://www.ehow.com/way_5332818_natural-ways-tighten-up-skin.html#ixzz26g3m3mxs

McMillan, T. (2011, July 5). Dangers of Bioflavonoids. http://www.livestrong.com/article/485460-dangers-of-bioflavonoids/

Meister, A. & Anderson, M.E. (1983). Glutathione. *Annual Review of Biochemistry.* 52: 711–6.

Meister, A. (1988). Glutathione metabolism and its selective modification. *The Journal of Biological Chemistry.* 263(33): 17205–8. http://www.jbc.org/content/263/33/17205.long

Meister, A. (1994). Glutathione-ascorbic acid antioxidant system in animals. *The Journal of Biological Chemistry.* 269(13): 9397–400. http://www.jbc.org/content/269/13/9397.long

Melissa. (2012, September 22). Personal communication.

Memorial Sloan-Kettering Cancer Center. (2005). About Herbs: Ellagic Acid. www.mskcc.org/mskcc/html/11571.cfm?RecordID=644&tab=HC

Mertens-Talcott, S.U. Lee, J.H., Percival, S.S. & Talcott, S.T. (2006). Induction of cell death in Caco-2 human colon carcinoma cells by ellagic acid rich fractions from muscadine grapes (Vitis rotundifolia). *Journal of Agricultural & Food Chemistry.* 54:5336-5343.

Meyer, A.S., Heinonen, M. & Frankel, E.N. (1998, January). Antioxidant interactions of catechin, cyanidin, caffeic acid, quercetin, and ellagic acid on human LDL oxidation. *Food Chemistry.* 61(1–2): 71–75.

Michaud, L. (2010, July 20). Copper Peptides Side Effects. http://www.livestrong.com/article/179847-copper-peptides-side-effects/

Miles, M.V. (2007, June). The uptake and distribution of coenzyme Q10. *Mitochondrion.* 7 (Suppl): S72–7.

Miller, E., Pastor-Barriuso, R., Dalal, D., Riemersma, R., Appel, L. & Guallar, E. (2005). Meta-analysis: high-dosage vitamin E supplementation may increase all-cause mortality. *Ann Intern Med.* 142(1): 37–46.

Miller, R.A., Harrison, D.E., Astle, C.M., Floyd, R.A., Flurkey, K., Hensley, K.L., Javors, M.A., Leeuwenburgh, C., Nelson, J.F., Ongini, E., Nadon, N.L., Warner, H.R. & Strong, R. (2007, August). An aging interventions testing program: Study design and interim report. *Aging Cell.* 6(4): 565–75.

Miranda. (2012, September 19). Personal communication.

Mokdad, A.H., Ford, E.S., Bowman, B.A., Dietz, W.H., Vinicor, F., Bales, V.S. & Marks, J.S. (2003). Prevalence of obesity, diabetes, and obesity-related health risk factors, 2001. *JAMA: the Journal of the American Medical Association.* 289(1): 76–9.

Montague, C.T., Farooqi, I.S., Whitehead, J.P., Soos, M.A., Rau, H., Wareham, N.J., Sewter, C.P., Digby, J.E., Mohammed, S.N., Hurst, J.A., Cheetham, C.H., Earley, A.R., Barnett, A.H., Prins, J.B. & O'Rahilly, S. (1997, June 26). Congenital leptin deficiency is associated with severe early-onset obesity in humans. *Nature.* 387(6636):903-8.

Montague, C.T. & O'Rahilly, S. (2000). The perils of portliness: Causes and consequences of visceral adiposity. *Diabetes.* 49(6): 883–8.

Moody, A.G. (2011, March 28). Does Apple Cider Vinegar Burn Body Fat? http://www.livestrong.com/article/23278-apple-cider-vinegar-burn-body/

Morie, R. (2012, May 26). How to Make Grapeseed Extract. http://www.ehow.com/how_5933210_make-grapeseed-extract.html

Moore, S. (Retrieved 2012). Bioflavonoids: Warnings & Side Effects. http://www.ehow.com/facts_5566048_bioflavonoids-warnings-side-effects.html

Moore, S. (2011, July 31). What Are the Dangers of Methylsulfonylmethane? http://www.livestrong.com/article/506314-what-are-the-dangers-of-methylsulfonylmethane/

Morris, D.L. & Rui, L. (2009). Recent advances in understanding leptin signaling and leptin resistance. *American Journal of Physiology, Endocrinology and Metabolism.* 297(6): E1247–59.

Mosha, T., Gaga, H., Pace, R., Laswai, H. & Mtebe, K. (1995). Effect of blanching on the content of antinutritional factors in selected vegetables. *Plant Foods Hum Nutr.* 47(4): 361–7.

Moskowitz, R.W. (2000, October). Role of collagen hydrolysate in bone and joint disease. *Semin. Arthritis Rheum.* 2:87-99.

Mozzon, M. (1996). Resveratrol content in some Tuscan wines. *Ital. J. Food Sci.* 8(2): 145–52. http://cat.inist.fr/?aModele=afficheN&cpsidt= 3123149

MSM Facts. (Retrieved 2012). http://www.kornax.com/Merchant2/MSM_Facts.htm

Mukhtar, H., Del Tito, B.J., Marcelo, C.L., Das, M. & Bickers, D.R. (1984). Ellagic acid: a potent naturally occurring inhibitor of benzo[a]pyrene metabolism and its subsequent glucuronidation, sulfation and covalent binding to DNA in cultured BALB/C mouse keratinocytes. *Carcinogenesis.* 5:1565-1571.

Muniyappa, R., Wong, K.A., Baldwin, H.L., Sorkin, J.D., Johnson, M.L., Bhasin, S., Harman, S.M. & Blackman, M.R. (2006). Dehydro-epiandrosterone secretion in healthy older men and women: effects of testosterone and growth hormone administration in older men. *J Clin Endocrinol Metab.* 91(11): 4445-4452.

Musa-Veloso, K., Card, J.W., Wong, A.W. & Cooper, D.A. (2009, September). Influence of observational study design on the interpretation of cancer risk reduction by carotenoids. *Nutr Rev.* 67(9):527-45.

Nahum, A., Sharoni, Y., Prall, O.W., Levy, J., Hirsch, K., Watts, C.K. & Danilenko, M. (2001). Lycopene inhibition of cell cycle progression in breast and endometrial cancer cells is associated with reduction in cyclin D levels and retention of p27(Kip1) in the cyclin E-cdk2 complexes. *Oncogene.* 20(26): 3428–436.

Nakamura, M. & Hayashi, T. (1994, June). One- and two-electron reduction of quinones by rat liver subcellular fractions. *J. Biochem.* 115(6): 1141–7.

Nall, R. (2011, June 14). Do Facial Exercises Really Tighten Skin? http://www.livestrong.com/article/294655-do-facial-exercises-really-tighten-skin/

Nalven, K. (Retrieved 2012). How to Boost Collagen Production & Firm Skin. http://www.ehow.com/how_6878194_boost-collagen-production-firm-skin.html

Narayanan, B.A. & Re, G.G. (2001). IGF-II down regulation associated cell cycle arrest in colon cancer cells exposed to phenolic antioxidant ellagic acid. *Anticancer Res.* 21:359-364.

Narisawa, T., Fukaura, Y., Hasebe, M., Ito, M., Nishino, H., Khachik, F., Murakoshi, M., Uemura, S. & Aizawa, R. (1996). Ihibitory effects of natural carotenoids, alpha-carotene, beta-carotene, lycopene and lutein, on colonic aberrant crypt foci formation in rats. *Cancer Lett.* 107(1): 137–142.

Nataloni, R. (2010, October 1). Fractional carbon dioxide lasers less invasive, but still carry risks. Cosmetic Surgery Times. http://www.modernmedicine.com/modernmedicine/Modern+Medicine+Now/Fractional-carbon-dioxide-lasers-less-invasive-but/ArticleStandard/Article/detail/688610

National Institutes of Health. (2011, April). DHEA: MedlinePlus Supplements. http://www.nlm.nih.gov/medlineplus/druginfo/natural/331.html

National Institutes of Health National Center for Complementary and Alternative Medicine. (Retrieved 2012). Herbs at a Glance: Aloe Vera. http://nccam.nih.gov/health/aloevera

National Institutes of Health Office of Dietary Supplements. (Retrieved 2012). Dietary Supplement Fact Sheet: Vitamin A. http://ods.od.nih.gov/factsheets/VitaminA-HealthProfessional/

National Institutes of Health Office of Dietary Supplements. (Retrieved 2012). Dietary Supplement Fact Sheet: Vitamin E. http://ods.od.nih.gov/factsheets/VitaminE-HealthProfessional//

Natural Guide to Skin Health. (Retrieved 2012). http://www.jashbotanicals.com/articles/natural_guide_skin_health_6.html

Navas, P., Villalba, J.M. & de Cabo, R. (2007, June). The importance of plasma membrane coenzyme Q in aging and stress responses. *Mitochondrion.* 7(Suppl): S34–40.

Nazarewicz, R.R., Ziolkowski, W., Vaccaro, P.S. & Ghafourifar, P. (2007). Effect of short-term ketogenic diet on redox status of human blood. *Rejuvenation Research.* 10(4): 435–40.

Nedergaard, J., Bengtsson, T. & Cannon, B. (2007). Unexpected evidence for active brown adipose tissue in adult humans. *AJP: Endocrinology and Metabolism.* 293(2): E444.

Nelson, L.R. & Bulun, S.E. (2001). Estrogen production and action. *Journal of the American Academy of Dermatology.* 45(3): S116–24.

Neporent, L. (2009, December 1). Exercises to Tighten Your Butt. http://www.thatsfit.com/2009/12/01/glute-butt-exercises

New Evidence That Caffeine Is a Healthful Antioxidant in Coffee. (2011, May 4). ScienceDaily. http://www.sciencedaily.com/releases/2011/05/110504095630.htm

Niki, E. (1987). Interaction of ascorbate and alpha tocopherol. *Third Conference on Vitamin C.* 498:187-98.

Nnama, H. (2010, November 11). Side Effects of Glucosamine Sulphate. http://www.livestrong.com/article/299461-side-effects-of-glucosamine-sulphate/

Non-Surgical Skin Tightening Treatments – More Hype Than Truth? (2011, May 6). http://www.medicalnewstoday.com/releases/224514.php

Nordberg, J. & Arner, E.S. (2001). Reactive oxygen species, antioxidants, and the mammalian thioredoxin system. *Free Radic Biol Med.* 31(11): 1287–312.

Norrish, A.E., Jackson, R.T., Sharpe, S.J. & Skeaff, C.M. (2000). Prostate cancer and dietary carotenoids. *Am J Epidemiol.* 151:119-123.

Novak, S. (2012). Eat 5 Green Foods to Improve Your Skin From the Inside Out. http://recipes.howstuffworks.com/green-foods-improve-skin.htm

Oakes, D. (2009, February 2). The Fountain of Youth Discovered: Rebounding: N.A.S.A. Approved Exercise. http://voices.yahoo.com/the-fountain-youth-discovered-2572259.html?cat=5

Oelke, E.A., Putnam, D.H., Teynor, T.M. & Oplinger, E.S. (1992, February). Quinoa. *Alternative Field Crops Manual.* University of Wisconsin Cooperative Extension. http://www.hort.purdue.edu/newcrop/afcm/quinoa.html

Ohkawara, K., Tanaka, S., Miyachi, M., Ishikawa-takata, K. & Tabata, I. (2007). A dose-response relation between aerobic exercise and visceral fat reduction: systematic review of clinical trials. *International Journal of Obesity (2005).* 31(12): 1786–1797.

Olas, B. & Wachowicz, B. (2005, August). Resveratrol, a phenolic antioxidant with effects on blood platelet functions. *Platelets.* 16(5): 251–60.

Olson, E.R., Naugle, J.E., Zhang, X., Bomser, J.A. & Meszaros, J.G. (2005, March). Inhibition of cardiac fibroblast proliferation and myofibroblast differentiation by resveratrol. *Am. J. Physiol. Heart Circ. Physiol.* 288(3): H1131–8.

Omenn, G., Goodman, G., Thornquist, M., Balmes, J., Cullen, M., Glass, A., Keogh, J., Meyskens, F., Valanis, B., Williams, J., Barnhart, S., Cherniack, M., Brodkin, C. & Hammar, S. (1996). Risk factors for lung cancer and for intervention effects in CARET, the beta-carotene and retinol efficacy trial. *J Natl Cancer Inst.* 88(21): 1550–9.

Onkst, T. (2011, June 14). How to Rebound for a Natural Face Lift. http://www.livestrong.com/article/306500-how-to-rebound-for-a-natural-face-lift/#ixzz26gCMEefl

Original Silicea Gel: A Natural Talent for Skin, Hair, and Fingernails. (Retrieved 2012). http://www.silicea.com/en/produkte/original_silicea_balsam.php

Ortega, R.M. (2006). Importance of functional foods in the Mediterranean diet. *Public Health Nutr.* 9(8A): 1136–40.

Padayatty, S.J., Katz, A., Wang, Y., Eck, P., Kwon, O., Lee, J., Chen, S., Corpe, C. *et al.* (2003). Vitamin C as an antioxidant: evaluation of its role in disease prevention. *Journal of the American College of Nutrition.* 22(1): 18–35. http://www.jacn.org/content/22/1/18.long

Paiva, S.A. & Russell, R.M. (1999). Beta-carotene and other carotenoids as antioxidants. *J Am Coll Nutr.* 18:426-433.

Palacios, A.I. (2010, August 14). The Effects of DHEA on Men. http://www.livestrong.com/article/204622-the-effects-of-dhea-on-men/

Palamara, A.T., Nencioni, L., Aquilano, K., De Chiara, G., Hernandez, L., Cozzolino, F., Ciriolo, M.R. & Garaci, E. (2005, May). Inhibition of influenza A virus replication by resveratrol. *J. Infect. Dis.* 191(10): 1719–29.

Palsamy, P. & Subramanian, S. (2008, November). Resveratrol, a natural phytoalexin, normalizes hyperglycemia in streptozotocin-nicotinamide induced experimental diabetic rats. *Biomed. Pharmacother.* 62(9): 598–605.

Pan, M.H. & Ho, C.T. (2008). Chemopreventive effects of natural dietary compounds on cancer development. *Chem Soc Rev.* 37(11): 2558–74.

Pankov, Y.A. (1999, June). Adipose tissue as an endocrine organ regulating growth, puberty, and other physiological functions. *Biochemistry (Mosc).* 64(6):601-9.

Pantuck, A.J., Leppert, J.T., Zomorodian, N., Aronson, W., Hong, J., Barnard, R.J., Seeram, N., Liker, H., Wang, H., Elashoff, R., Heber, D., Aviram, M., Ignarro, L. & Belldegrun, A. (2006). Phase II study of pomegranate juice for men with rising prostate-specific antigen following surgery or radiation for prostate cancer. *Clin Cancer Res.* 12:4018-4026. http://www.ncbi.nlm.nih.gov/pubmed/16818701

Paolini, M., Sapone, A. & Valgimigli, L. (2003, June). Avoidance of bioflavonoid supplements during pregnancy: a pathway to infant leukemia? *Mutat. Res.* 527(1–2): 99–101.

Papoutsi, Z., Kassi, E., Tsiapara, A., Fokialakis, N., Chrousos, G.P. & Moutsatsou, P. (2005). Evaluation of estrogenic/antiestrogenic activity of ellagic acid via the estrogen receptor subtypes ERalpha and ERbeta. *Journal of Agricultural & Food Chemistry*. 53:7715-7720.

Park, A. (2009, August 8). Fat-Bellied Monkeys Suggest Why Stress Sucks. *Time*. http://www.time.com/time/health/article/0,8599,1915237,00.html

Patterson, J. (2011, June 14). Why Low Potassium Causes Skin Problems. http://www.livestrong.com/article/287264-why-low-potassium-causes-skin-problems/

Peake, J. (2003). Vitamin C: effects of exercise and requirements with training. *Int J Sport Nutr Exerc Metab.* 13 (2): 125–51.

Pearson, O. (2011, May 14). Vitamins & Minerals for Connective Tissue. http://www.livestrong.com/article/442137-vitamins-minerals-for-connective-tissue/#ixzz25zwr1qci

Pearson, O. (2011, May 5). COQ10 & Foods. http://www.livestrong.com/article/435623-coq10-foods/

Pelleymounter, M.A., Cullen, M.J., Baker, M.B., Hecht, R., Winters, D., Boone, T. & Collins, F. (1995). Effects of the obese gene product on body weight regulation in ob/ob mice. *Science.* 269(5223): 540–3.

Pendergrass, T. (2011, May 26). Liver Detox & Cellulite. http://www.livestrong.com/article/328015-liver-detox-cellulite/

Penumathsa, S.V., Thirunavukkarasu, M., Zhan, L., Maulik, G., Menon, V.P., Bagchi, D. & Maulik, N. (2008, December). Resveratrol enhances GLUT-4 translocation to the caveolar lipid raft fractions through AMPK/Akt/eNOS signalling pathway in diabetic myocardium. *J. Cell. Mol. Med.* 12(6A): 2350–61.

Percival, M. (1998, June). Nutritional support for connective tissue repair and wound healing. *Clinical Nutrition Insights.* http://acudoc.com/Injury%20Healing.PDF

Perez-Meza, D., Leavitt, M. & Trachy, R. (1988). Clinical evaluation of GraftCyte moist dressings on hair graft viability and quality of healing. *Inter. J. Cos. Surg.* 6:80-84.

Perricone, N. (Retrieved 2012). What is CoQ10? The Benefits to Skin & Weight Loss. http://blog.perriconemd.com/what-is-coq10/

Perumal, S., Antipova, O. & Orgel, J. P. (2008). Collagen fibril architecture, domain organization, and triple-helical conformation govern its proteolysis. *PNAS.* 105 (8): 2824–2829.

Peters, U., Leitzmann, M.F., Chatterjee, N. *et al.* (2007). Serum lycopene, other carotenoids, and prostate cancer risk: A nested case-control study in the prostate, lung, colorectal, and ovarian cancer screening trial. *Cancer Epidemiol Biomarkers Prev.* 16: 962-968.

Pezeshkian, M., Noori, M., Najjarpour-Jabbari, H. *et al.* (2009, April). Fatty acid composition of epicardial and subcutaneous human adipose tissue. *Metab Syndr Relat Disord.* 7(2): 125–31

Pfefferle, W., Möckel, B., Bathe, B. & Marx, A. (2003). Biotechnological manufacture of lysine. *Advances in Biochemical Engineering/Biotechnology.* 79: 59–112.

Pharma Seeks Genetic Clues to Healthy Aging. (2010, April 6). *Reuters.* http://www.reuters.com/article/2010/04/06/us-age-genes-idUSTRE6350L620100406

Phytessence Wakame. (2009, January 7). http://www.truthinaging.com/ingredient-spotlight/phytessence-wakame-what-is-it

Pickart, L. (2008). The human tri-peptide GHK and tissue remodeling. *J. Biomater. Sci. Polymer Edn.* 19(8):969-988

Pickart, L., Freedman, J.H., Loker, W.J. *et al.* (1980). Growth-modulating plasma tripeptide may function by facilitating copper uptake into cells. *Nature.* 288(5792): 715–717.

Pickart, L. (Retrieved 2012). The Magic of Copper Peptides. http://www.copper-peptides.com/Science.html

Pilgeram, L. (2010). Control of fibrinogen biosynthesis, role of FFA/Albumin Ratio. *Cardiovasc Eng.* 10(2): 78–83.

Pilgeram, L. & Pickart, L. (1968). Control of fibrinogen biosynthesis, the role of free fatty acids. *J Atheroscler Res.* 8: 155–166.

Pitman, S. (2006, March 28). William Reed Business Media SAS. http://www.cosmeticsdesign.com/Formulation-Science/Research-suggests-glucosamine-is-an-effective-anti-aging-treatment

Pittler, M.H. & Ernst, E. (2006). Pittler, M.H., ed. Horse chestnut seed extract for chronic venous insufficiency. *Cochrane Database Syst Rev* (1): CD003230.

Pointel, J.P., Boccalon, H., Cloarec, M. *et al.* (1987). Titrated extract of Centella asiatica (TECA) in the treatment of venous insufficiency of the lower limbs. *Angiol.* 38:46-50.

Pollack, A., Madar, Z., Eisner, Z., Nyska, A. & Oren, P. (1997). Inhibitory effect of lycopene on cataract development in galactosemic rats. *Metab Pediatr Syst Ophthalmol.* 19(20): 31–36.

Pollard, J.D., Quan, S., Kang, T. & Koch, R.J. (2005). Effects of copper tripeptide on the growth and expression of growth factors by normal and irradiated fibroblasts. *Arch Facial Plast Surg.* 7(1):27-31.

Pond, C.M. (1998). *The Fats of Life.* Cambridge University Press.

Pool, R. (2001). *Fat: Fighting the Obesity Epidemic.* Oxford: Oxford University Press.

Porter, S.A., Massaro, J.M., Hoffmann, U., Vasan, R.S., O'Donnel, C.J. & Fox, C.S. (2009, June). Abdominal subcutaneous adipose tissue: a protective fat depot? *Diabetes Care.* 32(6):1068-75.

Poussier, B., Cordova, A.C., Becquemin, J.P. & Sumpio, B.E. (2005, December). Resveratrol inhibits vascular smooth muscle cell proliferation and induces apoptosis. *J. Vasc. Surg.* 42(6): 1190–7.

Prakash, S. *et al.* (2010). Role of coenzyme Q10 as an antioxidant and bioenergizer in periodontal diseases. *Indian J Pharmacol.* 42(6): 334–337.

Price, M.Z. (Retrieved 2012). Herbs That Tighten the Skin. http://www.ehow.com/about_5426838_herbs-tighten-skin.html

Prim. (2012, September 26). Personal communication.

Prior, R., Wu, X. & Schaich, K. (2005). Standardized methods for the determination of antioxidant capacity and phenolics in foods and dietary supplements. *J Agric Food Chem.* 53(10): 4290–302.

Procedures – Non-Surgical Skin Tightening (Thermage). (Retrieved 2012). http://www.cosmeticlaserskinsurgery.com/thermage.htm

Prokop, J., Abrman, P., Seligson, A.L. & Sovak, M. (2006). Resveratrol and its glycon piceid are stable polyphenols. *J Med Food.* 9(1): 11–4.

Proksch, E., Brandner, J.M. & Jensen, J.M. (2008). The skin: an indispensable barrier. *Exp Dermatol.* 17(12):1063–72.

Quirino, C. (2009, June 15). Potassium helps prevent itchy skin, pains. *Philippine Daily Inquirer.* http://showbizandstyle.inquirer.net/lifestyle/ lifestyle/view/20090615-210655/Potassium-helps-prevent-itchy-skin-pains

Raha, S. & Robinson, B.H. (2000). Mitochondria, oxygen free radicals, disease and ageing. *Trends in Biochemical Sciences.* 25(10): 502–8.

Rao, A.V. & Rao, L.G. (2007, March). Carotenoids and human health. *Pharmacol. Res.* 55(3): 207–16.

Raspanti, M., Ottani, V. & Ruggeri, A. (1990). Subfibrillar architecture and functional properties of collagen: a comparative study in rat tendons. *J Anat.* 172: 157–164.

Rattan, S. (2006). Theories of biological aging: genes, proteins, and free radicals. *Free Radic Res* 40 (12): 1230–8.

Reaume, A., Elliott, J., Hoffman, E., Kowall, N., Ferrante, R., Siwek, D., Wilcox, H., Flood, D., Beal, M., Brown, R., Scott, R. & Snider, W. (1996). Motor neurons in Cu/Zn superoxide dismutase-deficient mice develop normally but exhibit enhanced cell death after axonal injury. *Nat Genet.* 13 (1): 43–7.

Reference Guide for Amino Acids. (1995, October). http://www.realtime.net/anr/aminoacd.html

Reiter, R.J., Paredes, S.D., Manchester, L.C. & Tan, D. (2009). Reducing oxidative/nitrosative stress: A newly-discovered genre for melatonin. *Critical Reviews in Biochemistry and Molecular Biology.* 44 (4): 175–200.

Renaud, S. & de Lorgeril, M. (1992, June). Wine, alcohol, platelets, and the French paradox for coronary heart disease. *Lancet.* 339 (8808): 1523–6.

Restrepo, B. (2011, June 14). How to Get Rid of Cellulite Forever. http://www.livestrong.com/article/271673-how-to-get-rid-of-cellulite-forever/

Resveratrol. (Retrieved 2012). http://www.anyvitamins.com/resveratrol.htm

Resveratrol – How it Assists Skin and Connective Tissue Health. (Retrieved 2012). http://www.drsupplementreviews.com/health-center/resveratrol-assists-skin-and-connective-tissue-health.php

Resveratrol Side Effects. (Retrieved 2012). http://resveratrolsideeffectsexposed.com/

Resveratrol: Harvesting the Health Benefits of Spanish Red Wine Without the Alcohol. (2010). http://www.res-juventa.com

Reszko, A.E., Berson, D. & Lupo, M. (2009). Cosmeceuticals: practical applications. *Clinics in Dermatology*, 27(4):401-416.

Rhee, S., Chae, H. & Kim, K. (2005). Peroxiredoxins: a historical overview and speculative preview of novel mechanisms and emerging concepts in cell signaling. *Free Radic Biol Med*. 38(12): 1543–52.

Richmond, M. (Retrieved 2012). Home Cure for Loose and Sagging Skin. http://www.ehow.com/way_5721120_home-cure-loose-sagging-skin.html

Rietveld, A. & Wiseman, S. (2003). Antioxidant effects of tea: evidence from human clinical trials. *J Nutr*. 133(10): 3285S–3292S. http://jn.nutrition.org/content/133/10/3285S.full

Riles, W.L., Erickson, J., Nayyar, S., Atten, M.J., Attar, B.M. & Holian, O. (2006, September). Resveratrol engages selective apoptotic signals in gastric adenocarcinoma cells. *World J. Gastroenterol*. 12 (35): 5628–34.

Riley, S. (2009, June 25). Eating Superfoods for Health and Fitness. http://www.disabled-world.com/fitness/cooking/superfood.php#ixzz25STxgDx5

Rimas, A. (2006, December 11). His research targets the aging process. *The Boston Globe*. http://www.boston.com/news/globe/health_science/articles/2006/12/11/his_research_targets_the_aging_process/

Rimm, E.B., Stampfer, M.J., Ascherio, A., Giovannucci, E., Colditz, G.A. & Willett, W.C. (1993). Vitamin E consumption and the risk of coronary heart disease in men. *N Engl J Med*. 328(20): 1450–6.

Rippy, A. (2010, July 30). Exercises for Lifting & Firming Breasts With Extra Skin. http://www.livestrong.com/article/189049-exercises-for-lifting-firming-breasts-with-extra-skin/

Ristow, M., Zarse, K. & Oberbach, A. (2009). Antioxidants prevent health-promoting effects of physical exercise in humans. *Proc. Natl. Acad. Sci. U.S.A.* 106(21): 8665–70. http://www.ncbi.nlm.nih.gov/pmc/articles/PMC2680430/

Ristow, M. & Zarse, K. (2010). How increased oxidative stress promotes longevity and metabolic health: the concept of mitochondrial hormesis (mitohormesis). *Experimental Gerontology*. 45(6): 410–418.

Rizwan, M., Rodriguez-Blanco, I., Harbottle, A., Birch-Machin, M., Watson, R.E.B. & Rhodes, L.E. (2008, April 7-9). Lycopene protects against biomarkers of photodamage in human skin. *British Journal of Dermatology: Annual Meeting of the British Society for Investigative Dermatology*. 158, 4, 885-886.

Robb, E.L., Page, M.M., Wiens, B.E. & Stuart, J.A. (2008, March). Molecular mechanisms of oxidative stress resistance induced by resveratrol: Specific and progressive induction of MnSOD. *Biochem. Biophys. Res. Commun.* 367(2): 406–12.

Roberts, L.J., Oates, J.A. & Linton, M.F. (2007). The relationship between dose of vitamin E and suppression of oxidative stress in humans. *Free Radic. Biol. Med.* 43(10): 1388–93. http://www.ncbi.nlm.nih.gov/pmc/articles/PMC2072864/

Rodgers, G. (Retrieved 2012). How Amino Acids Help To Rejuvenate Your Skin. http://ezinearticles.com/?How-Amino-Acids-Help-To-Rejuvenate-Your-Skin&id=7071891

Rodriguez-Amaya, D. (2003). Food carotenoids: analysis, composition and alterations during storage and processing of foods. *Forum Nutr.* 56: 35–7.

Rohlandt, A. (2012). Skin Tightening Creams: Key Ingredients for Firmer Skin. http://www.dailyglow.com/skin-tightening-creams-key-ingredients-for-firmer-skin.html

Rousseau, N. (Retrieved 2012). How to Get Rid of Cellulite Forever: Transform Ugly Cellulite Into a Drop-Dead Gorgeous New You--Fast & Naturally. http://www.treatment-for-cellulite.com/

Roy, H. & Lundy, S. (2005). Resveratrol. *Pennington Nutrition Series, No. 7*. http://resveratrolpricewatch.com/PNS_Resveratrol.pdf

Ryo, K. *et al.* (2011, June). Effects of coenzyme Q10 on salivary secretion. *Clin Biochem.* 44(8-9):669-74.

Sage, E.H. & Gray, W.R. (1977). Evolution of elastin structure. *Adv. Exp. Med. Biol.* 79: 291–312.

Sahelian, R. (Retrieved 2012). Collagen Supplements, Benefit and Side Effects, Dosage and Type. http://www.raysahelian.com/collagen.html

Salamone, M. (2011, October 15). Manganese and Skin Health. http://mauriziosalamone.blogspot.com/2011/10/manganese-and-skin-health.html

Sandberg, A. (2002). Bioavailability of minerals in legumes. *Br J Nutr.* 88 (Suppl 3): S281–5.

Santos, A.C., Veiga, F. & Ribeiro, A.J. (2011, August). New delivery systems to improve the bioavailability of resveratrol. *Expert Opin Drug Deliv.* 8(8): 973–90.

Sarao, C. (2010, May 16). How to Repair Skin Cellulite. http://www.livestrong.com/article/124404-repair-skin-cellulite/#ixzz25e5Mg200

Sareen, D., van Ginkel, P.R., Takach, J.C., Mohiuddin, A., Darjatmoko, S.R., Albert, D.M. & Polans, A.S. (2006, September). Mitochondria as the primary target of resveratrol-induced apoptosis in human retinoblastoma cells. *Invest. Ophthalmol. Vis. Sci.* 47 (9): 3708–16.

Schlesinger, D.H., Pickart, L. & Thaler, M.M. (1977). Growth-modulating serum tripeptide is glycyl-histidyl-lysine. *Cellular and Molecular Life Sci.* 33(3): 324–325.

Schmatz, R., Mazzanti, C.M., Spanevello, R., Stefanello, N., Gutierres, J., Corrêa, M., da Rosa, M.M., Rubin, M.A., Chitolina Schetinger, M.R. & Morsch, V.M. (2009,

May). Resveratrol prevents memory deficits and the increase in acetylcholinesterase activity in streptozotocin-induced diabetic rats. *Eur. J. Pharmacol.* 610(1–3): 42–8.

Schmelzer, C., Kubo, H., Mori, M. *et al.* (2010, June). Supplementation with the reduced form of Coenzyme Q10 decelerates phenotypic characteristics of senescence and induces a peroxisome proliferator-activated receptor-alpha gene expression signature in SAMP1 mice. *Mol Nutr Food Res.* 54(6): 805–15.

Schmidt, P.J., Daly, R.C., Bloch, M., Smith, M.J., Danaceau, M.A., St Clair, L.S., Murphy, J.H., Haq, N. & Rubinow, D.R. (2005). Dehydro-epiandrosterone monotherapy in midlife-onset major and minor depression. *Arch Gen Psychiatry.* 62.2 154-162.

Schneider, C. (2005). Chemistry and biology of vitamin E. *Mol Nutr Food Res.* 49(1): 7–30.

Schocker, L. (2012, April 25). Surprisingly Calcium-Rich Foods That Aren't Milk. *The Huffington Post.* http://www.huffingtonpost.com/ 2012/04/25/calcium-food-sources_n_1451010.html

Schuler, L., Forsythe, C. & Cosgrove, A. (2007). *The New Rules of Lifting for Women: Lift Like a Man, Look Like a Goddess.* Avery Publishers.

Schulz, T.J., Zarse, K., Voigt, A., Urban, N., Birringer, M. & Ristow, M. (2007). Glucose restriction extends Caenorhabditis elegans life span by inducing mitochondrial respiration and increasing oxidative stress. *Cell Metab.* 6(4): 280–93.

Schumacker, P. (2006). Reactive oxygen species in cancer cells: Live by the sword, die by the sword. *Cancer Cell.* 10 (3): 175–6.

Schwarz, D. & Roots, I. (2003, April). In vitro assessment of inhibition by natural polyphenols of metabolic activation of procarcinogens by human CYP1A1. *Biochem. Biophys. Res. Commun.* 303(3): 902–7.

Sea Buckthorn: A True Super Food for Health and Beauty. (2012). http://applesanddoctors.com/sea-buckthorn-a-true-super-food

Sea Buckthorn Oil Side Effects. (Retrieved 2012). http://www.buzzle.com/articles/sea-buckthorn-oil-side-effects.html

Seaver, L.C. & Imlay, J.A. (2004). Are respiratory enzymes the primary sources of intracellular hydrogen peroxide? *Journal of Biological Chemistry.* 279(47): 48742–50.

Seeram, N.P., Adams, L.S., Henning, S.M. *et al.* (2005, June). In vitro antiproliferative, apoptotic and antioxidant activities of punicalagin, ellagic acid and a total pomegranate tannin extract are enhanced in combination with other polyphenols as found in pomegranate juice. *J. Nutr. Biochem.* 16(6): 360–7.

Seifried H., McDonald, S., Anderson, D., Greenwald, P. & Milner, J. (2003). The antioxidant conundrum in cancer. *Cancer Res.* 63 (15): 4295–8. http://cancerres.aacrjournals.org/content/63/15/4295.full

Seiler, A., Schneider, M., Förster, H., Roth, S., Wirth, E.K., Culmsee, C., Plesnila, N., Kremmer, E. *et al.* (2008). Glutathione peroxidase 4 senses and translates oxidative stress into 12/15-lipoxygenase dependent- and AIF-mediated cell death. *Cell Metabolism*. 8(3): 237–48.

Selenium. (Retrieved 2012). http://www.whfoods.com/genpage.php?dbid=95&tname=nutrient

Sen, C.K., Khanna, S. & Roy, S. (2006). Tocotrienols: Vitamin E beyond tocopherols. *Life Sciences*. 78 (18): 2088–98. http://www.ncbi.nlm.nih.gov/pmc/articles/PMC1790869/

Seo, H.J., Cho, Y.E, Kim, T., Shin, H.I., Kwun, I.S., Seo, H.J., Cho, Y.E., Kim, T., Shin, H.I. & Kwun, I.S. (2010, October) Zinc may increase bone formation through stimulating cell proliferation, alkaline phosphatase activity and collagen synthesis in osteoblastic MC3T3-E1 cells. *Nutr Res Pract*. 4(5):356-61.

Sesso, H.D., Buring, J.E. & Christen, W.G. (2008). Vitamins E and C in the prevention of cardiovascular disease in men: the Physicians' Health Study II randomized controlled trial. *JAMA*. 300(18): 2123–33. http://www.ncbi.nlm.nih.gov/pmc/articles/PMC2586922/

Seward, Z.M. (2006, November 30). Quest for youth drives craze for 'wine' pills. *The Wall Street Journal*. http://www.post-gazette.com/pg/06334/742471-114.stm

Shayan, R., Achen, M.G. & Stacker, S.A. (2006). Lymphatic vessels in cancer metastasis: bridging the gaps. *Carcinogenesis*. 27(9): 1729–38.

Shenkin, A. (2006). The key role of micronutrients. *Clin Nutr*. 25 (1): 1–13.

Shin, M.H., Rhie G.E., Park C.H., Kim K.H., Cho K.H., Eun H.C. & Chung J.H. (2005, February). Modulation of collagen metabolism by the topical application of dehydroepiandrosterone to human skin. *J Invest Dermatol*. 124(2):315-23.

Shock – Some Collagen Repair Skin Treatments Actually Work. (2008, May 28). *Scientific Blogging*. http://www.science20.com/news_releases/shock_some_collagen_repair_skin_treatments_actually_work

Shukla A, Rasik, A.M., Jain, G.K. *et al*. (1999). In vitro and in vivo wound healing activity of asiaticoside isolated from Centella asiatica. *J Ethnopharmacol*. 65:1-11.

Side Effects of Retinol A. (Retrieved 2012). http://www.ehow.com/about_4682331_side-effects-retinol.html

Sies, H. (1993). Strategies of antioxidant defense. *European Journal of Biochemistry*. 215(2): 213–9.

Sies, H. (1997). Oxidative stress: Oxidants and antioxidants. *Experimental Physiology*. 82(2): 291–5.

Signs and Symptoms of Cellulite. (Retrieved 2012). http://www.homeremediesweb.com/cellulite_home_remedy.php

Sikorski, Z.E. (2001). *Chemical and Functional Properties of Food Proteins*. Boca Raton: CRC Press.

Siméon, A., Emonard, H., Hornebeck, W. & Maquart, F.X. (2000). The tripeptide-copper complex glycyl-L-histidyl-L-lysine-Cu2+ stimulates matrix metalloproteinase-2 expression by fibroblast cultures. *Life Sci*. 22,67(18):2257-65

Siméon, A., Wegrowski, Y., Bontemps, Y. & Maquart, F.X. (2001). Expression of glycosaminoglycans and small proteoglycans in wounds: modulation by the tripeptide-copper complex glycyl-L-histidyl-L-lysine-Cu(2+). *J Invest Dermatol.* 115(6):962-8

Sirtori, C.R. (2001, September). Aescin: pharmacology, pharmacokinetics and therapeutic profile. *Pharmacol. Res.* 44(3): 183–193.

Sirtris Announces Positive Results with Proprietary Version of Resveratrol, SRT501, in a Phase 1b Type 2 Diabetes Clinical Study - Drugs.com MedNews. (2008, January 1). http://www.drugs.com/clinical_trials/sirtris-announces-positive-results-proprietary-version-resveratrol-srt501-phase-1b-type-2-diabetes-3127.html

Skin Brushing. (Retrieved 2012). http://www.jashbotanicals.com/articles/skin_brushing.html

Skin Tightening Options. (Retrieved 2012). http://www.healthyskinportal.com/skin-tightening.cfm

Skin Tightening Using Radiofrequency or Pulsed Light. (Retrieved 2012). http://www.surgery.org/consumers/procedures/skin/non-surgical-skin-tightening

Slideshow: Cellulite Pictures, Causes, Myths, and Treatments. (2012, March 14). http://www.webmd.com/healthy-beauty/ss/slideshow-cellulite-pictures-causes-myths-and-treatments

Smirnoff, N. (2001). L-Ascorbic acid biosynthesis. *Vitamins and Hormones.* 61: 241–66.

Smirnoff, N. & Wheeler, G.L. (2000). Ascorbic acid in plants: Biosynthesis and function. *Critical Reviews in Biochemistry and Molecular Biology.* 35(4): 291–314.

Smith, E. (2011, August 18). How to Tighten the Skin With Mustard Oil. http://www.livestrong.com/article/516636-how-to-tighten-the-skin-with-mustard-oil/#ixzz26OzGhJ8i

Sohal, R. (2002). Role of oxidative stress and protein oxidation in the aging process. *Free Radic Biol Med.* 33(1): 37–44.

Sohal, R., Mockett, R. & Orr, W. (2002). Mechanisms of aging: an appraisal of the oxidative stress hypothesis. *Free Radic Biol Med.* 33(5): 575–86.

Sorenson, J.R.J., Soderberg, L.S.F. & Chang, L.W. (1995). Radiation protection and radiation recovery with essential metalloelement chelates, *Proc. Soc. Exper. Biol. And Med.* 210: 191 – 204.

Spalding, K.L., Arner, E., Westermark, P.O., Bernard, S., Buchholz, B.A., Bergmann, O., Blomqvist, L., Hoffstedt, J. *et al.* (2008). Dynamics of fat cell turnover in humans. *Nature.* 453(7196): 783–7.

Stadtman, E. (1992). Protein oxidation and aging. *Science.* 257(5074): 1220–4.

Stahl, W. & Sies, H. (1996). Lycopene: a biologically important carotenoid for humans? *Arch. Biochem. Biophys.* 336(1): 1–9.

Staker, L. (2011, August 9). Ways to Promote Lymphatic Drainage. http://www.livestrong.com/article/511819-ways-to-promote-lymphatic-drainage/#ixzz261DCTOa0

Stanner, S.A., Hughes, J., Kelly, C.N. & Buttriss, J. (2004). A review of the epidemiological evidence for the 'antioxidant hypothesis.' *Public Health Nutr.* 7(3): 407–22.

Staton, M. (Retrieved 2012). Skin Firming & Thickening Oral Supplements. http://www.ehow.com/list_6625363_skin-firming-thickening-oral-supplements.html

Stefani, M., Markus, M.A., Lin, R.C., Pinese, M., Dawes, I.W. & Morris, B.J. (2007, October). The effect of resveratrol on a cell model of human aging. *Ann. N. Y. Acad. Sci.* 1114: 407–18.

Steinhardt, E., Israeli, C. & Lambert, R.A. (1913). Studies on the cultivation of the virus of vaccinia. *J. Inf Dis.* 13, 294–300.

Stipanuk, M.H. & Caudill, M.A. (2006). *Biochemical, Physiological and Molecular Aspects of Human Nutrition.* Saunders.

Stipp, D. (2007, January 19). Can red wine help you live forever? *Fortune.* http://money.cnn.com/2007/01/18/magazines/fortune/Live_forever.fortune/index.htm?postversion=2007011912

Stohs, S.J. & Bagchi, D. (1995). Oxidative mechanisms in the toxicity of metal ions. *Free Radic. Biol. Med.* 18(2): 321–36.

Stokes, B. (2010, May 26). Solutions for Loose Skin on Thighs. http://www.livestrong.com/article/131667-solutions-loose-skin-thighs/

Stone, B. (Retrieved 2012). How to Firm Face Skin Naturally. http://www.dailyglow.com/how-to-firm-face-skin-naturally.html

Stoppani, J. (2010, January). *Muscle & Fitness Presents 2010 Edition: The Ultimate Supplement Handbook.* http://www.muscleandfitness.com/features/other/ultimate-supplement-handbook

Strous, R.D., Maayan, R., Lapidus, R., Stryjer, R., Lustig, M., Kotler, M. & Weizman, A. (2003, February). Dehydroepiandrosterone augmentation in the management of negative, depressive, and anxiety symptoms in schizophrenia. *Arch Gen Psychiatry.* 60(2):133-41.

Study Citing Antioxidant Vitamin Risks Based On Flawed Methodology, Experts Argue. (2007, March 1). Oregon State University. http://www.sciencedaily.com/releases/2007/02/070228172604.htm

Suh, J.M., Zeve, D., McKay, R., Seo, J., Salo, Z., Li, R., Wang, M. & Graff, J.M. (2007). Adipose is a conserved dosage-sensitive antiobesity gene. *Cell Metabolism.* 6(3): 195–207.

Sundstrom, K. (2011, May 25). Vitamins & Minerals Needed to Keep Skin Firm. http://www.livestrong.com/article/454015-vitamins-minerals-needed-to-keep-skin-firm/

Sweeney, S. M. *et al.* (2008). Candidate Cell and Matrix Interaction Domains on the Collagen Fibril, the Predominant Protein of Vertebrates. *J Biol Chem.* 283(30): 21187–21197.

Szmitko, P.E. & Verma, S. (2005, January). Cardiology patient pages. Red wine and your heart. *Circulation.* 111(2): e10–1.

Szpak, P. (2011). Fish bone chemistry and ultrastructure: implications for taphonomy and stable isotope analysis. *Journal of Archaeological Science*. 38(12): 3358–3372.

Takanami, Y., Iwane, H., Kawai, Y. & Shimomitsu, T. (2000). Vitamin E supplementation and endurance exercise: are there benefits? *Sports Med*. 29(2): 73–83.

Tanzi, E. (2011, August 24). Skin Tightening: Surgical vs. Non-Surgical. http://www.doctoroz.com/blog/elizabeth-tanzi-md/skin-tightening-surgical-vs-non-surgical

Tapia, P. (2006). Sublethal mitochondrial stress with an attendant stoichiometric augmentation of reactive oxygen species may precipitate many of the beneficial alterations in cellular physiology produced by caloric restriction, intermittent fasting, exercise and dietary phytonutrients: Mitohormesis for health and vitality. *Medical Hypotheses*. 66(4): 832–43.

Taylor, L.L. (Retrieved 2012). Skin Disorders - Can Fish Oil Omega3 Improve Skin Health? http://www.articlecity.com/articles/health/article_7681.shtml

Tchoukalova, Y.D., Votruba, S.B., Tchkonia, T., Giorgadze, N., Kirkland, J.L. & Jensen, M.D. (2010). Regional differences in cellular mechanisms of adipose tissue gain with overfeeding. *PNAS*. 107(42): 18226–31.

Teichert, J. & Preiss, R. (1992). HPLC-methods for determination of lipoic acid and its reduced form in human plasma. *International Journal of Clinical Pharmacology, Therapy, and Toxicology*. 30(11): 511–2.

Tennen, R.I., Michishita-Kioi, E. & Chua, K.F. (2012, February). Finding a target for resveratrol. *Cell*. 148(3): 387–9.

The Beauty Benefits of Green Tea. (Retrieved 2012). http://www.ivillage.co.uk/the-beauty-benefits-green-tea/76175

The Coffee Enema for Liver Detoxification. (Retrieved 2012). http://curezone.com/art/read.asp?ID=28&db=5&C0=818

The Doctor Within: Collagen Supplement. (Retrieved 2012). http://www.thedoctorwithin.com/collagen/Collagen/

The Dubious Practice of Detox. (Retrieved 2012). http://www.health.harvard.edu/healthbeat/HEALTHbeat_072208.htm#art1

The Healthy Skin Benefits of Lycopene. (Retrieved 2012). http://www.causesandremedies.com/the-healthy-skin-benefits-of-lycopene/

The Secrets of Beautiful Skin: Discover the Benefits of Fish Oil for Skin. (Retrieved 2012). http://www.thesecretsofbeautifulskin.com/discover-the-benefits-of-fish-oil-for-skin.html

The Skin Benefits of Green Tea Extract. (2011, March 20). http://skincareclub.wordpress.com/2011/03/20/skin-benefits-green-tea-extract/

Thermage® Thermalift Skin Tightening. (Retrieved 2012). http://www.lasersurgery.com/thermage/

Thomas, D. (2004). Vitamins in health and aging. *Clin Geriatr Med*, 20(2): 259–74.

Thorne Research Inc. (2003). Methylsulfonylmethane (MSM). *Alternative Medicine Review*, 8, 4: 438-441. http://www.altmedrev.com/publications/8/4/438.pdf

Thorne Research, Inc. (2009). Aesculus hippocastanum (Horse chestnut). *Alternative Medicine Review.* Volume 14, Number 3. http://www.thorne.com/altmedrev/fulltext/14/3/278.pdf

Thresiamma, K.C., George, J. & Kuttan, R. (1998). Protective effect of curcumin, ellagic acid and bixin on radiation induced genotoxicity. *J Exp Clin Cancer Res.* 17:431-434.

Tighten and Firm Loose or Saggy Body Skin. (Retrieved 2012). http://www.outsidehealth.net/product-p/ohi11.htm

Tiidus, P. (1998). Radical species in inflammation and overtraining. *Can J Physiol Pharmacol.* 76(5): 533–8. http://www.nrcresearchpress.com/doi/abs/10.1139/y98-047

Titan, M. (Retrieved 2012). How Does Rebounding Get Rid of Cellulite? http://ezinearticles.com/?How-Does-Rebounding-Get-Rid-of-Cellulite?&id=1664902

Tiu, M. (Retrieved 2012). Foods for Beautiful Healthy Skin. http://ezinearticles.com/?Foods-For-Beautiful-Healthy-Skin&id=2853963

Today's Woman. (Retrieved 2012). Beauty – Free Face Exercises. http://www.todays-woman.co.uk/free-face-exercises.shtml

Todorov, G. (Retrieved 2012). Can coenzyme Q10 help protect and repair your skin? http://www.smartskincare.com/treatments/topical/coq10.html

Todorov, G. (Retrieved 2012). Copper Peptides - Can You Repair a Wrinkle? http://www.smartskincare.com/treatments/topical/copper.html

Top 10 Foods Highest in Copper. (Retrieved 2012). http://www.healthaliciousness.com/articles/high-copper-foods.php

Traber, M.G. & Atkinson, J. (2007). Vitamin E, antioxidant and nothing more. *Free Radical Biology and Medicine.* 43 (1): 4–15. http://www.ncbi.nlm.nih.gov/pmc/articles/PMC2040110/

Tran, W. (2008, May 5). Dry Skin Brushing Improves The Lymph System. http://www.holistichealthlibrary.com/dry-skin-brushing-and-the-lymph-system/

Trantas, E., Panopoulos, N. & Ververidis, F. (2009, November). Metabolic engineering of the complete pathway leading to heterologous biosynthesis of various flavonoids and stilbenoids in Saccharomyces cerevisiae. *Metab. Eng.* 11(6): 355–66.

Traub, W., Yonath, A. & Segal, D. M. (1969). On the molecular structure of collagen. *Nature.* 221(5184): 914–917.

Travis, W. (Retrieved 2012). Am I a Candidate for IPL Photofacial? http://www.healthyskinportal.com/articles/photofacial-candidate/178/

Trentham, D., Dynesius-Trentham, R., Orav, J., Combitchi, D., Lorenzo, C., Sewell, K., Hafler, D. & Weiner, H. (1993). Effects of oral administration of type II collagen on rheumatoid arthritis. *Science.* 261(5119): 1727–1730.

Turcotte, M. (2009, November 3). Foods That Have Ellagic Acid. http://www.livestrong.com/article/70095-foods-ellagic-acid/#ixzz267GxPf00

Turunen, M., Olsson, J. & Dallner, G. (2004). Metabolism and function of coenzyme Q. *Biochimica et Biophysica Acta.* 1660(1–2): 171–99.

U.S. Food and Drug Administration. (2009, July 9). 187 Fake Cancer 'Cures' Consumers Should Avoid. http://www.fda.gov/Drugs/GuidanceCompliance RegulatoryInformation/EnforcementActivitiesbyFDA/ucm171057.htm

Ullmann, M. (Retrieved 2012). Amino Acid Skin Care. www.ehow.com/facts_ 6038798_amino-acid-skin-care.html

University of Maryland Medical Center: Alpha Lipoic Acids. (2011). http://www.umm.edu/altmed/articles/alpha-lipoic-000285.htm

University of Maryland Medical Center: Amino Acids. (2011). http://www.umm.edu/ency/article/002222.htm

University of Maryland Medical Center: Beta-Carotene. (2011). http://www.umm.edu/altmed/articles/beta-carotene-000286.htm

University of Maryland Medical Center: Calcium. (2011). http://www.umm.edu/altmed/articles/calcium-000290.htm

University of Maryland Medical Center: Coenzyme Q10. (2011). http://www.umm.edu/altmed/articles/coenzyme-q10-000295.htm

University of Maryland Medical Center: Copper. (2011). http://www.umm.edu/altmed/articles/copper-000296.htm

University of Maryland Medical Center: Creatine. (2011). http://www.umm.edu/altmed/articles/creatine-000297.htm

University of Maryland Medical Center: Cysteine. (2011). http://www.umm.edu/altmed/articles/cysteine-000298.htm

University of Maryland Medical Center: Docosahexaenoic Acid (DHA). (2011). http://www.umm.edu/altmed/articles/docosahexaenoic-acid-000300.htm

University of Maryland Medical Center: Glucosamine. (2011). http://www.umm.edu/altmed/articles/glucosamine-000306.htm

University of Maryland Medical Center: Glutamine. (2011). http://www.umm.edu/altmed/articles/glutamine-000307.htm

University of Maryland Medical Center: Gotu Kola. (2011). http://www.umm.edu/altmed/articles/gotu-kola-000253.htm

University of Maryland Medical Center: Grape Seed. (2011). http://www.umm.edu/altmed/articles/grape-seed-000254.htm

University of Maryland Medical Center: Green Tea. (2011). http://www.umm.edu/altmed/articles/green-tea-000255.htm

University of Maryland Medical Center: Horsetail. (2011). http://www.umm.edu/altmed/articles/horsetail-000257.htm

University of Maryland Medical Center: Hyaluronic Acid. (2011). http://www.umm.edu/drug/notes/Hyaluronic-acid-On-the-skin.htm

University of Maryland Medical Center: Carnitine (L-Carnitine). (2011). http://www.umm.edu/altmed/articles/carnitine-l-000291.htm

University of Maryland Medical Center: Lysine. (2011). http://www.umm.edu/altmed/articles/lysine-000312.htm

University of Maryland Medical Center: Manganese. (2011). http://www.umm.edu/altmed/articles/manganese-000314.htm

University of Maryland Medical Center: Omega 3 Fatty Acids. (2011). http://www.umm.edu/altmed/articles/omega-3-000316.htm

University of Maryland Medical Center: Phenylalanine. (2011). http://www.umm.edu/altmed/articles/phenylalanine-000318.htm

University of Maryland Medical Center: Quercetin. (2011). http://www.umm.edu/altmed/articles/quercetin-000322.htm

University of Maryland Medical Center: Selenium. (2011). http://www.umm.edu/altmed/articles/selenium-000325.htm

University of Maryland Medical Center: Tryptophan. (2011). http://www.umm.edu/ency/article/002332.htm

University of Maryland Medical Center: Tyrosine. (2011). http://www.umm.edu/altmed/articles/tyrosine-000329.htm

University of Maryland Medical Center: Vitamin B-2 (Riboflavin). (2011). http://www.umm.edu/altmed/articles/vitamin-b2-000334.htm

University of Maryland Medical Center: Vitamin B-3 (Niacin). (2011). http://www.umm.edu/altmed/articles/vitamin-b3-000335.htm

University of Maryland Medical Center: Vitamin B-6 (Pyridoxine). (2011). http://www.umm.edu/altmed/articles/vitamin-b6-000337.htm

University of Maryland Medical Center: Vitamin C (Ascorbic Acid). (2011). http://www.umm.edu/altmed/articles/vitamin-c-000339.htm

University of Maryland Medical Center: Vitamin C. (2011). http://www.umm.edu/ency/article/002404all.htm

University of Maryland Medical Center: Vitamin E. (2011). http://www.umm.edu/altmed/articles/vitamin-e-000341.htm

University of Maryland Medical Center: Zinc. (2011). http://www.umm.edu/altmed/articles/zinc-000344.htm

University of Milano, Department of Pharmacological Sciences. (2001, September). Aescin: pharmacology, pharmacokinetics and therapeutic profile. *Sirtori CR*, 44(3):183-93.

University of Rochester Medical Center. (2008, March 26). Mounting Evidence Shows Red Wine Antioxidant Kills Cancer. http://www.urmc.rochester.edu/news/story/index.cfm?id=1934

Uno, H. & Kurata, S. (1993, July). Chemical agents and peptides affect hair growth. *J Invest Dermatol.* 101(1 Suppl):143S-147S

Uscher, J. (Retrieved 2012). Nutrients for Healthy Skin. http://www.webmd.com/healthy-beauty/features/skin-nutrition

Using Hyaluronic Acid for Skin Care. (Retrieved 2012). http://www.ivlproducts.com/Health-Library/Health-Concerns/Anti-Aging/Using-Hyaluronic-Acid-for-Skin-Care/

Uzoma, K. (2011, June 14). Percentage of Americans who diet every year. http://www.livestrong.com/article/308667-percentage-of-americans-who-diet-every-year/
Vaccariello, L. (2010, April 9). 8 Foods for Younger-Looking, Supple Skin. NBC Today Show. http://today.msnbc.msn.com/id/36273089/ns/today-today_health/t/foods-younger-looking-supple-skin/
Vaishampayan, U., Hussain, M., Banerjee, M., Seren, S., Sarkar, F.H., Fontana, J., Forman, J.D., Cher, M.L., Powell, I., Pontes, J.E. & Kucuk, O. (2007). Lycopene and soy isoflavones in the treatment of prostate cancer. *Nutr Cancer.* 59:1-7.
Valenzano, D.R., Terzibasi, E., Genade, T., Cattaneo, A., Domenici, L. & Cellerino, A. (2006, February). Resveratrol prolongs lifespan and retards the onset of age-related markers in a short-lived vertebrate. *Curr. Biol.* 16(3): 296–300.
Valko, M., Morris, H. & Cronin, M.T. (2005). Metals, toxicity and oxidative stress. *Curr. Med. Chem.* 12(10): 1161–208.
Valko, M., Leibfritz, D., Moncol, J., Cronin, M., Mazur, M. & Telser, J. (2007). Free radicals and antioxidants in normal physiological functions and human disease. *The International Journal of Biochemistry & Cell Biology.* 39(1): 44–84.
Valko, M., Izakovic, M., Mazur, M., Rhodes, C.J. & Telser, J. (2004). Role of oxygen radicals in DNA damage and cancer incidence. *Molecular and Cellular Biochemistry.* 266(1–2): 37–56.
Van Camp, W., Inzé, D. & Van Montagu, M. (1997). The regulation and function of tobacco superoxide dismutases. *Free Radic Biol Med.* 23(3): 515–20.
van de Poll, M.C., Dejong, C.H. & Soeters, P.B. (2006). Adequate range for sulfur-containing amino acids and biomarkers for their excess: lessons from enteral and parenteral nutrition. *J. Nutr.* 136(6 Suppl): 1694S–1700S.
Van Gaal, L., Mertens, I. & De Block, C. (2006). Mechanisms linking obesity with cardiovascular disease. *Nature.* 444(7121): 875–80.
Van Marken Lichtenbelt, W.D., Vanhommerig, J.W., Smulders, N.M., Drossaerts, J.M., Kemerink, G.J., Bouvy, N.D., Schrauwen, P. & Teule, G.J. (2009). Cold-activated brown adipose tissue in healthy men. *The New England Journal of Medicine.* 360(15): 1500–8.
Vanaman, B. (2010, February 24). Dangers of L-Carnitine. http://www.livestrong.com/article/86784-dangers-lcarnitine/
Vanaman, B. (2011, July 17). What Are the Benefits of Seaweed Extract for Arthritis? http://www.livestrong.com/article/494761-what-are-the-benefits-of-seaweed-extract-for-arthritis/
Vattem, D.A. & Shetty, K. (2005, June 30). Biological function of ellagic acid: A review. *Journal of Food Biochemistry.* 29(3): 234-266.
Vertuani, S., Angusti, A. & Manfredini, S. (2004). The antioxidants and pro-antioxidants network: An overview. *Current Pharmaceutical Design.* 10(14): 1677–94.
Vieira Dos Santos, C. & Rey, P. (2006). Plant thioredoxins are key actors in the oxidative stress response. *Trends Plant Sci.* 11(7): 329–34.

Villareal, D.T. & Holloszy, J.O. (2004). Effect of DHEA on abdominal fat and insulin action in elderly women and men: a randomized controlled trial. *JAMA.* 292(18): 2243-2248.
Virgili, F. & Marino, M. (2008). Regulation of cellular signals from nutritional molecules: a specific role for phytochemicals, beyond antioxidant activity. *Free Radical Biology & Medicine.* 45(9): 1205–16.
Virtanen, K.A., Lidell, M.E., Orava, J., Heglind, M., Westergren, R., Niemi, T., Taittonen, M., Laine, J. *et al.* (2009). Functional brown adipose tissue in healthy adults. *The New England Journal of Medicine.* 360(15): 1518–25.
Vitamin C Serum Side Effects. (Retrieved 2012). http://healthbeautyandskincare products.com/vitamin-c-serum-side-effects
Vivekananthan, D.P., Penn, M.S., Sapp, S.K., Hsu, A. & Topol, E.J. (2003). Use of antioxidant vitamins for the prevention of cardiovascular disease: meta-analysis of randomised trials. *Lancet.* 361 (9374): 2017–23.
Vogel, G. & Ströcker, H. (1966, December 16). The effect of drugs--especially flavonoids and aescin--on the lymph flow and the permeability of the intact plasma-lymph barrier of rats for fluid and defined macromolecules. *Arzneimittelforschung.* (12):1630-4. http://www.ncbi.nlm.nih.gov/pubmed/6014798
Voorhees, J.J., Fisher G.J. & Varani, J. (2008). Looking Older: Fibroblast Collapse and Therapeutic Implications. *Archives of Dermatology. 144:5.*
Wada, H., Goto, H., Hagiwara, S. & Yamamoto, Y. (July 2007). Redox status of coenzyme Q10 is associated with chronological age. *J Am Geriatr Soc.* 55(7): 1141–2.
Wade, N. (2006, November 16). Red Wine Ingredient Increases Endurance, Study Shows. *New York Times.* http://www.nytimes.com/2006/11/17/health/17iht-web.1117wine.3582746.html?_r=1
Wagner, B. (2011, May 3). Dry Skin Brushing – How To Do. http://wagnerhealthcare.wordpress.com/2011/05/03/dry-skin-brushing-how-to-do/
Waistline Worries: Turning Apples Back Into Pears. http://www.healthywomen. org/columns/drpeekescolumn/dbcolumn/waistlineworriesturningapplesbackinto pears
Walle, T., Hsieh, F., DeLegge, M.H., Oatis, J.E. & Walle, U.K. (2004, December). High absorption but very low bioavailability of oral resveratrol in humans. *Drug Metab. Dispos.* 32(12): 1377–82.
Wang, D. (2011, August 11). Exercises to Tighten Up Sagging Skin on the Chin. http://www.livestrong.com/article/91244-exercises-tighten-up-sagging-skin/
Ward, J. (1998). Should antioxidant vitamins be routinely recommended for older people? *Drugs Aging.* 12(3): 169–75.
Washington, I. (Retrieved 2012). What Can Collagen Supplements Do for Skin? http://www.ehow.com/about_5509957_can-collagen-supplements-do-skin.html

Wegrowski, Y., Maquart, F.X. & Borel, J.P. (1992). Stimulation of sulfated glycosaminoglycan synthesis by the tripeptide-copper complex glycyl-L-histidyl-L-lysine-Cu2+. *Life Sci.* 51(13): 1049-56.

Weintraub, A. (2009, July 29). Resveratrol: The hard sell on anti-aging. *Bloomberg Businessweek.* http://www.businessweek.com/magazine/content/09_32/b4142000175800.htm

Welbourne, T.C. (1995). Increased plasma bicarbonate and growth hormone after an oral glutamine load. *The American Journal of Clinical Nutrition.* 61(5): 1058-1061.

Wenzel, E. & Somoza, V. (2005, May). Metabolism and bioavailability of trans-resveratrol. *Mol Nutr Food Res.* 49(5): 472–81.

Wess, T.J., et al. (1998). Molecular packing of type I collagen in tendon. *J Mol Biol.* 275(2): 255–267.

Whitney, N. (Retrieved 2012). How to Boost the Collagen in Your Skin. http://www.ehow.com/how_5643243_boost-collagen-skin.html

Why Use Antioxidants? (2007, February 11). http://www.specialchem4adhesives.com/tc/antioxidants/index.aspx?id=

Widgerow, A.D., Chait, L.A., Stals, R. & Stals, P.J. (2000). New innovations in scar management. *Aesthetic Plast Surg.* 24:227-34.

William Reed Business Media SAS. (2004, September 2). Beta-Carotene Boosts Skin Health, Suggests Study. http://www.nutraingredients.com/Research/Beta-carotene-boosts-skin-health-suggests-study

Williams, R.J., Spencer, J.P. & Rice-Evans, C. (2004). Flavonoids: antioxidants or signalling molecules? *Free Radical Biology & Medicine.* 36(7): 838–49.

Wilson, J. & Gelb, A. (2002). Free radicals, antioxidants, and neurologic injury: possible relationship to cerebral protection by anesthetics. *J Neurosurg Anesthesiol.* 14(1): 66–79.

Wilson, R. (1995). *Aromatherapy for Vibrant Health & Beauty/ A Practical A to Z Reference of Aromatherapy Treatments for Health, Skin, and Hair Problems Using Essential Oils.* Avery.

Witschi, A., Reddy, S., Stofer, B. & Lauterburg, B. (1992). The systemic availability of oral glutathione. *Eur J Clin Pharmacol.* 43(6): 667–9.

Wolf, G. (2005). The discovery of the antioxidant function of vitamin E: The contribution of Henry A. Mattill. *The Journal of Nutrition.* 135(3): 363–6.

Wolff, J.D. (Retrieved 2012). Risks of Collagen Supplements. http://www.ehow.com/about_4743039_risks-collagen-supplements.html

Wong, C. (2012, September 19). What You Need to Know About DHEA/DHEA Side Effects and Safety: What Should You Know About It? http://altmedicine.about.com/od/dhea/a/dhea.htm

Wong, C. (2012, September 20). Grape Seed Extract: What Should I Know About It? http://altmedicine.about.com/od/completeazindex/a/grapeseed.htm

Wong, C. (2011, September 26). Can Collagen Supplements Improve Your Skin? http://altmedicine.about.com/od/skinconditions/a/Collagen-Skin.htm

Wong, C. (2012, September 15). Fucoxanthin: What Is Fucoxanthin? http://altmedicine.about.com/od/herbsupplementguide/a/fucoxanthin.htm

Wood, J.G., Rogina, B., Lavu, S., Howitz, K., Helfand, S.L., Tatar, M. & Sinclair, D. (2004, August). Sirtuin activators mimic caloric restriction and delay ageing in metazoans. *Nature.* 430(7000): 686–9.

Wood, Z., Schröder, E., Robin Harris, J. & Poole L. (2003). Structure, mechanism and regulation of peroxiredoxins. *Trends Biochem Sci.* 28(1): 32–40.

Woodside, J., McCall, D., McGartland, C. & Young, I. (2005). Micronutrients: dietary intake v. supplement use. *Proc Nutr Soc.* 64(4): 543–53.

Worwood, V.A. (1991). *The Complete Book of Essential Oils and Aromatherapy.* New World Library.

Wu, G., Fang, Y.Z., Yang, S., Lupton, J.R. & Turner, N.D. (2004). Glutathione metabolism and its implications for health. *J. Nutr.* 134(3): 489–92.

Wyckoff, R., Corey, R. & Biscoe, J. (1935). X-ray reflections of long spacing from tendon. *Science.* 82(2121): 175–176.

Yan, X., Chuda, Y., Suzuki, M. & Nagata, T. (1999). Fucoxanthin as the major antioxidant in Hijikia fusiformis, a common edible seaweed. *Bioscience, Biotechnology and Biochemistry.* 63(3): 605-607.

Záková, P., Kanďár, R., Skarydová, L., Skalický, J., Myjavec, A. & Vojtísek, P. (2007, May). Ubiquinol-10/lipids ratios in consecutive patients with different angiographic findings. *Clin. Chim. Acta.* 380(1-2): 133–8.

Zalet. (2009, August 4). Resveratrol sources. http://www.zalet.com/resveratrol-sources-resveratrol-red-grapes-juice/

Zeibig, J., Karlic, H., Lohninger, A., Dumsgaard, R. & Smekal, G. (2005, September). Do blood cells mimic gene expression profile alterations known to occur in muscular adaption in enduranced training? *European Journal of Applied Physiologics.* 95: 96-104.

Zingg, J. & Azzi, A. (2004). Non-antioxidant activities of vitamin E. *Current Medicinal Chemistry.* 11(9): 1113–33.

Zita, Č., Overvad, K., Mortensen, S.A., Sindberg, C.D., Moesgaard, S. & Hunter, D.A. (2003). Serum coenzyme Q10concentrations in healthy men supplemented with 30 mg or 100 mg coenzyme Q10 for two months in a randomised controlled study. *BioFactors.* 18(1–4): 185–93.

Zold, E., Szodoray, P., Gaal, J., Kappelmayer, J., Csathy, L., Gyimesi, E., Zeher, M., Szegedi, G. & Bodolay, E. (2008, October 18). Vitamin D deficiency in undifferentiated connective tissue disease. *Arthritis Research & Therapy.* 10:R123 http://arthritis-research.com/content/10/5/R123

About the Author

Melynda Majors spends most of her free time obsessing about weight loss and the rest obsessing over basset hounds. She currently is managed and directed by one basset hound, William, and one affectionate 20½ pound orange tabby cat, BOB. Both are rescues.

Melynda holds a bachelor's degree from Rollins College and a master's degree from Florida State University. Originally from Orrville, Alabama, she lives and works in Washington, D.C.

After years of composing essays, speeches, reports, non-profit grant applications and various other yawn-inspiring written pieces, this is her first full-length book.

Final Thoughts

Learn more about firming loose skin at
www.firmlooseskin.com

Shop for the supplements, extracts, equipment and other items mentioned in this book online at
http://astore.amazon.com/firlooski-20

Top 5 Tips to Firm Your Skin:

Take your vitamins!
Lift heavy weights!
Jump on a rebounder!
Dry brush your skin!
Drink your water!

Made in the USA
Las Vegas, NV
22 February 2021